T0189387

Case Studies in
Medicine for the Elderly

Case Studies in Medicine for the Elderly

S.C. Allen

BSc, MD, MRCP,
Consultant Physician in Medicine for the Elderly,
Christchurch Hospital, Dorset

D.S. Fairweather

MA, PhD, MRCP,
Consultant Physician and Clinical Lecturer in Geriatric Medicine
at the University of Oxford and The Radcliffe Infirmary, Oxford

J.C. Brocklehurst

MSc, MD, FRCP,
Professor of Geriatric Medicine, University of Manchester

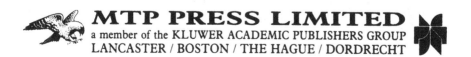

MTP PRESS LIMITED
a member of the KLUWER ACADEMIC PUBLISHERS GROUP
LANCASTER / BOSTON / THE HAGUE / DORDRECHT

Published in the UK and Europe by
MTP Press Limited
Falcon House
Lancaster, England

British Library Cataloguing in Publication Data

Allen, S.C.
    Case studies in medicine for the elderly.
    1. Geriatrics
    I. Title II. Fairweather, D.S.
    III. Brocklehurst, J.C.
    618.97   RC952

    ISBN 0-85200-698-5

Published in the USA by
MTP Press
A division of Kluwer Academic Publishers
101 Philip Drive
Norwell, MA 02061, USA

Library of Congress Cataloging-in-Publication Data

Allen, S.C. (Stephen C.)
    Case studies in medicine for the elderly.

    Bibliography: p.
    Includes index.
    1. Geriatrics--Case studies. I. Fairweather, D.S.,
1948-   . II. Brocklehurst, J.C. (John Charles)
III. Title. [DNLM: 1. Geriatrics--problems. WT 18 A429c]
RC952.7.A44 1987   618.97'0076   87-2913
ISBN 0-85200-698-5

Printed and bound in Great Britain by Anchor Brendon,
Tiptree, Essex

CONTENTS

PREFACE

This book is not intended to be a comprehensive textbook of medicine in old age. We have, however, aimed to present the reader with a collection of clinical problems typical of the scope of work in a department of medicine for the elderly. The questions are laid out as a medley of multiple-choices, short answers, data interpretations and discussions which will be of value to those preparing for a number of examinations, such as the Diploma in Geriatric Medicine, Membership of the Royal College of Physicians and Membership of the Royal College of General Practitioners. Undergraduates will also find the book useful as a supplementary reader for geriatric medicine and general internal medicine.

We accept that some of the answers given are contentious; this is inevitable in any book of this type, and is particularly so when the subject is as diverse and rapidly growing as geriatric medicine. The reader who wishes to expand upon a topic is advised to refer to the reading list at the end of the book which has been chosen to include a range of differing styles and approaches to the subject. Also, a short list of suggested further reading is given at the end of each case study.

We convey our thanks to the editorial staff of MTP Press for their advice during the later stages of production of the book, to the Department of Medical Illustration at The University Hospital of South Manchester, and to Sue Whitworth for typing the manuscript.

S C Allen
D S Fairweather
J C Brocklehurst

CASE 1

DECLINING MOBILITY

HISTORY

A lady of 70 years of age was admitted to a geriatric unit so that her husband could have a one week rest from looking after her. She had become progressively less mobile over the preceding 6 months, and at the time of admission was virtually bedbound. She had suffered from osteoarthrosis of the hips, knees and ankles for several years and her family doctor had attributed the decline to her present immobile state to worsening of her degenerative joint disease. She mentioned a 2-week history of urinary incontinence; she was unaware of passing urine, but found her clothes saturated with urine when she came to change. On direct questioning she admitted that her legs had become weaker in recent months, and that she had noticed some numbness of the right foot. She had a 15-year history of hypertension; her surgical history included a hysterectomy for uterine fibroids, and traumatic dislocation of the left hip, both many years ago. Before admission she was taking methyldopa, bendrofluazide and aspirin, all of which were continued after her admission.

Question A

Which of the following statements are correct?

1. The patient's generalised osteoarthrosis is likely to be a significant factor in her declining mobility.

2. The urinary incontinence is probably caused by a urinary tract infection.

3. A detailed neurological examination is likely to yield useful diagnostic information.

4. The progressive history of her condition is misleading.

5. The description of the urinary incontinence suggests a neurological cause.

EXAMINATION

She was moderately obese, compos mentis and in good spirits. Her blood pressure was 190/105 mmHg. On examination, the cardiovascular system, chest and abdomen were normal, though she had a large amount of firm stool in the rectum. Her cranial nerves and speech were normal. Both legs were hypertonic, with ankle clonus, though the tone in the arms was normal. Muscle power was reduced

1

to MRC grade 4 in extension, abduction and adduction, and grade 3 in flexion of the right hip, grade 2 in flexion and extension of the right knee and grade 0 in dorsiflexion of the right ankle. Power loss was very slight in the muscles of the left leg. Sensory testing revealed absence of light touch, vibration and proprioception below the T12 dermatome bilaterally, and reduction in pain, deep pressure and temperature sensation in the same distribution. The optic fundi were normal. There was painless bony enlargement of both knees and crepitus was felt over the patellae when the knees were flexed and extended; moderate painless limitation of flexion of the knees and hips was found.

Question B

Discuss:

1. How are the grades of muscle power defined in the MRC 0-5 classification?

2. How does muscle power grading give useful information in this patient?

3. At what anatomical level is the lesion probably situated?

Question C

Which of the following are correct?

1. A lumbar puncture will probably yield diagnostic biochemical abnormalities.

2. Lumbar myelography should be performed.

3. The natural history of the patient's condition should be observed for a further month before investigations are arranged.

4. Radiographs of the dorsal and lumbar spine should be examined.

5. Nerve conduction studies should be performed before treatment.

Question D

Discuss:

Are any other investigations likely to provide evidence of the anatomical site of the lesion?

INVESTIGATIONS

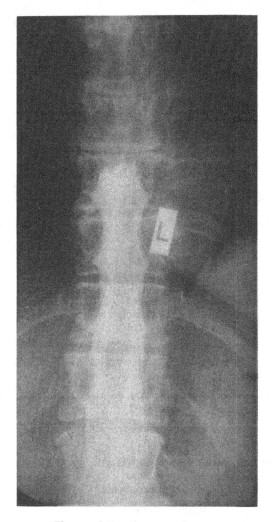

Figure 1 Lumbar myelogram

Question E

Discuss:

What are the abnormal features on these radiographs (Figures 1 and 2)? Name the lesions which could cause these appearances.

What is the differential diagnosis of spastic paraparesis?

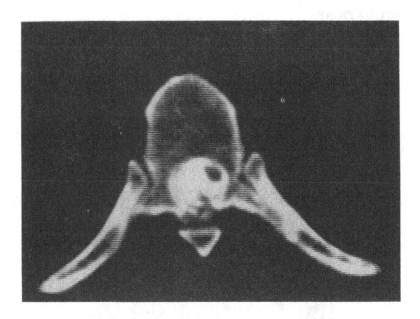

Figure 2 CT radiograph at the level of D10 taken immediately after the myelogram

Question F

In view of the patient's symptoms, signs and radiological abnormalities would you:

1. Begin intensive physiotherapy to try to restore the patient to her previous level of mobility?

2. Arrange neurosurgical decompression of her spinal cord as soon as possible?

3. Transfer the patient to a continuing care (long stay) ward on the grounds that no treatment can be offered to a patient of this age with a spastic paraparesis?

4. Delay surgical treatment until progression of the lesion has been demonstrated clinically?

5. Try a course of electrical spinal cord stimulation before resorting to a major surgical decompression procedure?

MANAGEMENT

At operation a spinal meningioma at the D8-10 level was almost completely removed and the weakness of her legs began to improve within a few days. She was transferred from the neurosurgical ward to the geriatric rehabilitation ward.

Question G

Which of the following is likely to be true of her further progress?

1. The remaining fragment of meningioma will grow and begin compressing the spinal cord within a few months.

2. A urinary catheter should be left in situ until no further neurological improvement is observed.

3. Physiotherapy has little to offer in the patient's postoperative rehabilitation.

4. Her osteoarthrosis could become the main barrier to her becoming independent in walking.

5. Postural hypotension might occur when she starts walking again.

ANSWERS

Question A   1, 3 and 5 are correct.

Although the patient's degenerative joint disease may not be the main reason for her recent deterioration, it will certainly exacerbate it; the unsteadiness which results from stiff, painful and deformed joints is exaggerated in the presence of pain, weakness or disequilibrium from other causes.

Urinary tract infection is more often a consequence of urinary incontinence than a cause of it, though incontinence may be more difficult to treat when the urinary tract is infected, particularly when urgency is a feature.

It is essential to perform a complete neurological examination to define the nature of the patient's weakness; sensory examination will help determine the likely site of a neurological lesion, and must include testing of perineal sensation in a patient with incontinence, particularly when bladder sensation has been lost.

The progressive history is not misleading; it indicates that a steadily advancing pathology is the likely cause of the patient's problems, rather than pathology of sudden onset such as stroke, spinal cord infarction or trauma.

The uncontrolled passing of urine of which the patient is unaware **always** signifies a neurological cause; the lesion may be in the sensory nerves of the bladder itself, the cauda equina, the sacral "bladder centre" or the spinal cord (see case 29).

Question B

1. Muscle power grading:

    0 = no movement

    1 = a flicker of muscle movement, but not enough to move the joint

    2 = can move the part, but not against gravity

3 = can move the part against gravity

4 = less than full power

5 = full power, allowing for age, sex and build

2.   Muscle power grading, though fairly crude, allows a semi-quantitative record of muscle power to be made; thus changes over time can be more reliably followed. This is particularly important when deciding whether a neurological lesion is progressive or not. Elderly patients frequently misjudge the degree of muscle weakness, so an objective record becomes doubly important. Of course, power grading must always be interpreted alongside examination of muscle tone, reflexes and sensation, and within the context of the patient's symptoms.
      Grading the power in this patient highlights the pattern of weakness; it emphasises the lower limb weakness and the observation of normal power in the upper limbs is important. Baseline power grading will allow the effects of treatment to be assessed.

3.   In the lower thoracic/lumbar region the anatomical site of a lesion will be about 3 higher than its dermatome value; therefore, as the level of this patient's sensory dermatome abnormality is T12, the lesion will be approximately at the level of the 9th thoracic vertebra.

Question C   2 and 4 are correct.

The measurement of CSF pressure may indicate a dynamic spinal block (Queckenstedt test positive) and the CSF chemistry may be abnormal; in this patient the CSF protein was raised to 1.08 g/l (normal 0.25-0.75 g/l). However, this is found in a number of spinal cord diseases (e.g. tumour, demyelination, infection) and is by no means diagnostic.
      It would not be wise to observe the patient for longer as this might delay surgical treatment to the extent that the chances of eventual recovery are greatly reduced.
      Radiographs of the thoracic and lumbar spines are an essential first step to rule out spinal disease, which may be encroaching upon the spinal cord, either directly or due to vertebral collapse, such as myeloma, metastatic carcinoma, osteoporosis, osteomalacia, tuberculosis, pyogenic abscess or Paget's disease. A prolapsed intervertebral disc cannot be diagnosed on a single plain radiograph in elderly patients. Cord compression must be considered in all undiagnosed cases of spastic paraparesis.
      Lumbar myelography will demonstrate the site, size and shape of the lesion, and is particularly useful when a lesion is compressing or expanding the spinal cord. A myelogram can cause worsening of transverse myelitis and should be avoided if that condition is thought to be present.

Question D

Computed tomography of the thoracic and lumbar areas, particularly when combined with lumbar myelography yields useful information on the site, size, shape and to a certain extent, the composition of a lesion compressing or expanding the spinal cord.

Question E

Myelogram There is a complete myelographic block at D10 with displacement of the spinal cord to the left. The subarachnoid space is widened on the right; the features are those of an intradural extramedullary tumour. There are also degenerative changes present in the lumbar spine.

Computerised tomogram The tumour is seen lying on the right posterolateral aspect of the spinal cord. The lesion is most likely to be a meningioma. These appearances could also be caused by a neurofibroma.

The differential diagnosis of a spastic paraparesis includes spinal cord trauma, cord demyelination, transverse myelitis, subacute combined degeneration of the spinal cord, intramedullary tumours (glioma, ependymoma, parasaggital cranial meningioma and anterior spinal artery thrombosis).

Question F   2 is correct.

Only surgical removal of the tumour can offer any hope of improving the patient's spinal cord function. This should be arranged urgently once the diagnosis is established; delaying could result in a total irreversible loss of cord function. There is no evidence that electrical spinal cord stimulation aids recovery, and it should certainly not be contemplated as an alternative to surgery. To transfer an otherwise well patient with a potentially treatable lesion to a long-stay ward would be very poor geriatric practice indeed.

Question G   4 and 5 are correct.

This patient's lower limb strength improved to such an extent that the main reason why several weeks of rehabilitation were required was that her osteoarthrotic hips and knees were very stiff and painful. Postoperatively, physiotherapy was by far the most important aspect of her rehabilitation; she needed only a minimal amount of occupational therapy to become independent in the activities of daily living (ADL).

Postural hypotension is often encountered when an elderly patient starts walking again after a prolonged period of immobility; it is occasionally a major obstacle in rehabilitation. This patient had continued to receive methyldopa to control her supine blood pressure; this drug was stopped and the postural hypotension resolved.

Meningiomata grow slowly, recurrence of compression is unlikely to occur, and a patient of this age is likely to succumb to other pathology meanwhile.

The urinary catheter was removed as soon as the patient had recovered from the operation itself; thereby bladder filling could occur and the patient was able to start experiencing the sensation of a full bladder as soon as sensory function began to recover. This facilitated the relearning of bladder control and hence continence of urine was soon achieved. Keeping the urinary catheter in until sensory recovery was complete would have delayed this process.

An elderly patient whose mobility is declining to an extent which is greater than that which normally occurs in old age requires careful clinical evaluation, investigation, treatment and, often, rehabilitation.

Suggested further reading

Pathy M S F (1985) The central nervous system - clinical presentation and management of neurological disorders in old age. In: Brocklehurst J C (ed.) Textbook of Geriatric Medicine and Gerontology, 3rd Edn. Churchill Livingstone, Edinburgh

Schlick H, Stille D (1975) Clinical symptomatology of intraspinal tumors. In: Vinken P J and Brugn G W (eds.) Handbook of Clinical Neurology, Vol. 19: Tumors of the spine and spinal cord, North-Holland, Amsterdam

CASE 2

FALLS - 1

PRESENTATION

A 79-year-old retired headmistress presented to Casualty at 5.00 pm on a Sunday afternoon. She lived alone in a bungalow, and had consulted her GP six times in the previous ten days because of falls. The ambulance had been called when the patient's daughter learned that she had fallen again earlier in the day. The neighbour noticed that the patient was a little confused at times. In the past she had suffered from mild hypertension and osteoarthrosis but had been generally in good health. She was taking moduretic, 1 tab/day, α-methyldopa, 250 mg tds, nitrazepam, 10 mg at night, ibuprofen, 400 mg tds and quinine sulphate, 600 mg at night. Over the last few months she had been feeling vaguely unwell and had lost about one stone in weight; she had also been suffering from headaches and constipation. Her falls had only started recently and occurred at night, while getting up to pass urine, or in the early morning. The casualty officer could find nothing obviously wrong on examination, and wished to discharge her, but both the patient and her daughter refused, insisting that she was not able to manage alone; the registrar in geriatric medicine was then called.

Question A

Which of the following are true about depression in the elderly?

1. Claims of ill-health, in the absence of abnormal physical signs, are likely to be functional.

2. Attention-seeking behaviour is common in those living alone.

3. Proven weight loss always has an organic cause.

4. Agitation and depression commonly co-exist.

5. A physically frail subject is unlikely to commit suicide.

EXAMINATION

She was weeping; blood pressure 100/60 mmHg lying and standing; shortened R.C.P. mental test score 10/10 (score of 7/10 or less suggestive of dementia); she had an unsteady gait, but no focal neurological signs and there was no evidence of fracture.

Question B

Which of the following do you think are reasonable statements?

9

1. The falls are probably due to "drop-attacks".

2. The falls are probably due to vertebrobasilar ischaemia secondary to cervical spondylosis.

3. You should do an urgent ESR in view of the headaches and weight loss.

4. Hyponatraemia may be present as the patient is taking moduretic.

5. There is nothing abnormal to find but you will admit the patient for tests.

TREATMENT AND PROGRESS

A careful history by the admitting doctor established:

1. The patient had been "low" for about six months, feeling that life was not worth living. Her appetite had been poor, the bowels sluggish and she had difficulty doing her normal chores. She also had difficulty in sleeping and wept often. All this was out of character.

2. The falls had started shortly after she was prescribed nitrazepam for her insomnia.

The hypotension persisted, and the α-methyldopa was stopped, though a diuretic was continued since she had an enlarged heart on her chest radiograph, and a tendency to oedema (the ECG showed left bundle branch block). After this the blood pressure was stable at 160/90 mmHg.

Other tests were:

Hb 9.8 g/dl; MCV 84 fl; MCH 26.7 pg; MCHC 32 g/dl, serum Fe 9 μmol/l;
TIBC 40 μmol/l; ESR 65 mm/h; RA latex and SCAT negative.
Radiographs of her hands showed an erosive arthropathy with destruction of the radial head and ulnar styloid; those of her knees showed severe degenerative changes.

No falls occurred after stopping the hypnotic and hypotensive agents. A psychogeriatrician's opinion was that she was severely depressed and should be treated with a tetracyclic antidepressant. It was felt that active rheumatoid arthritis (erosive arthropathy and anaemia of chronic disease), α-methyldopa and possible nitrazepam, were contributing to her depression.

Question C

Which of the following may occur while taking nitrazepam?

1. Confusion/disorientation

2. Dysarthria

3. Blurred vision

4.   Falls

5.   Rebound wakefulness

Question D

Which of the following benzodiazepines always have a plasma elimination half-life less than 24 hours in old people?

1.   Nitrazepam

2.   Diazepam

3.   Temazepam

4.   Flurazepam

5.   Lorazepam

DISCUSSION AND ANSWERS

Question A   4 is correct.

Depression is not uncommon among the elderly, and untangling the contribution from the depression itself from that due to associated physical disease is a major challenge for the physician. Depressed patients are not immune from physical illness, and physical complaints should be taken seriously.   Hypochondriasis and attention-seeking behaviour are more likely to be long-standing personality traits than to appear for the first time in an elderly subject. Weight loss is common among severely depressed patients and special attention may have to be paid to their calorie intake. Agitation may be a presenting feature of depression.   Suicide may be attempted by patients of any age, including those who are very dependent.

Question B   4 is correct.

There is insufficient information on which to diagnose the cause of her falls. Drop attacks can be diagnosed only with a clear history, and it is uncommon for falls to be directly attributable to cervical spondylosis. No clear diagnostic features of giant cell arteritis have been   given   to   justify   an   emergency   ESR,   but   significant hyponatraemia is not uncommon among elderly diuretic-takers, and is possibly more common in those taking moduretic.   Although this patient needs to be admitted, it would be wrong to conclude that nothing abnormal has been found. Old people do not cry without reason, and a blood pressure of 100/60 mmHg is rather low at this age and suggests she is being over-treated with hypotensive agents.

Question C   1, 2, 3 and 4 are correct.

These are the main side-effects of nitrazepam,   and of benzodiazepines in general, in the elderly. Rebound wakefulness is more

likely to occur during therapy with very short-acting benzodiazepines, but may occur upon stopping any hypnotic. It is likely
that this patient suffered from confusion and falls due to the hypnotic. She only began to fall after it was prescribed and did not fall
again after it was stopped. It is probable that the unsteadiness
observed on admission was due to accumulation of nitrazepam.

Question D   None correct.

Except temazepam, all these drugs can have long half-lives in young
subjects - in the case of flurazepam up to four days. Among the
old, half-life is either unchanged or prolonged. In the case of
temazepam, the half-life in the young is between 5 and 10 hours,
but in the old may be prolonged to over a day. This has been
shown to result in sufficient accumulation to interfere with afternoon performance after one week's treatment.

Suggested further reading

Abramowicz M (ed.) (1981) Choice of benzodiazepines. Medical Letter on Drugs and
Therapeutics, **23**, 41-42

Neshkes R E, Jarvik L F (1985) The central nervous system - dementia and delirium in
old age. In: Brocklehurst J C (ed.) Textbook of Geriatric Medicine and Gerontology.
Churchill Livingstone, Edinburgh

Overstall P W (1984) Hypnotics. In: O'Malley K (ed.) Clinical Pharmacology and Drug
Treatment in the Elderly. Churchill Livingstone, Edinburgh

CASE 3

FALLS AND CONFUSION - 1

HISTORY

A 90-year-old lady was admitted to hospital with a one week history of falls. She had been sensible and well orientated up to the time of admission. Twelve months previously she had suffered sudden bilateral loss of vision; a diagnosis of giant cell arteritis was made and she was treated with prednisolone, though her vision did not improve. She was taking nitrazepam, 5 mg at night up to the time of admission. Her elderly husband, who was disabled by chronic respiratory failure, had been admitted to another hospital one week prior to her admission.

Question A

True or false?

1. Most elderly blind people fall at least once a week.

2. Blindness caused by giant cell arteritis usually improves when steroid therapy is given.

3. The use of temazepam rather than nitrazepam as a hypnotic in elderly patients eliminates the risk of falls caused by benzo-diazepine hangover.

4. Giant cell arteritis occurs very infrequently in the 9th and 10th decades.

5. The treatment of giant cell arteritis in extreme old age requires about half the dose of prednisolone that is given to patients in the 65-75 age group.

6 HOURS AFTER ADMISSION

Later on the day of admission she became acutely confused and thought she was in a church. She was anxious and restless, and became incontinent of urine, apparently for the first time. She was afebrile, and there were no changes on physical examination, other than a mild tachycardia of 110/min. Her vision was of light/dark discrimination only; it was noted that her hearing aid had no battery.

Question B

Discuss:
1. What is the most likely reason for her acute confusion?

2. Which investigations will give useful clinical information at this stage?

Question C

Acute confusion in elderly patients is frequently observed in:

1. B_{12} deficiency anaemia

2. Upper gastrointestinal haemorrhage

3. Atrial fibrillation

4. Pneumonia

5. Hypertension

INVESTIGATIONS AT THE TIME OF THE ACUTE CONFUSION

Hb 13.2 g/dl; WCC 8.2 x 10^9/l with a normal differential;
ESR 22 mm/h; chest radiograph normal; ECG normal;
Na 136 mmol/L; K 3.4 mmol/l; urea 6.2 mmol/l; glucose 8.0 mmol/l.

Question D

Discuss:

Are the results above of any help in the diagnosis of this patient?

Question E

Discuss:

How would you manage the patient initially?

Question F

Discuss:

How can further episodes of the same nature be avoided?

Question G

Which of the following are true about acute confusion?

1. It is commoner in women.

2. Formed delusions are a major feature.

3. Mania is usually indistinguishable.

4. It can be caused by a stroke.

5. All medications should always be stopped upon admission to hospital.

ANSWERS

Question A   All are false.

Blind people do not fall often, even in old age. When an elderly blind patient is falling, it is essential to search for other causes,

14

though poor vision may be compounding the problem.

The blindness of giant cell arteritis often occurs suddenly, though there are usually preceding symptoms, such as headache, transient visual disturbances or symptoms of polymyalgia rheumatica. Vision rarely returns when corticosteroid treatment is given, hence the need to make an early diagnosis and start treatment before visual loss occurs. Giant cell arteritis probably occurs as often in the 80+ group as in the 70-80 age group. Very elderly patients should receive corticosteroid treatment at the same dosage as younger patients.

Though temazepam, triazolam and other short half-life hypnotics are less likely than nitrazepam to cause hangover drowsiness the next day, this is not to be relied upon in elderly patients, some of whom excrete such drugs quite slowly.

Question B

This is a good example of acute confusion due to sensory deprivation; the patient had virtually no visual or auditory input, but she was remaining orientated in her own home where the daily routine, odours, objects and people were familiar. These all disappeared upon her admission to hospital, so she quickly became disorientated, confused and anxious.

A reasonable approach to the initial investigation in this patient is to arrange for Hb, WBC count, chest radiograph, ECG, urea, electrolytes and blood glucose to rule out some of the more common causes of acute confusion in old patients.

When confused patients are febrile, a urine microscopy and culture, and blood cultures must be performed. Arterial blood gas tensions should be measured when acutely confused patients have signs of heart failure or respiratory disease.

Question C   2 and 4

Patients with B_{12} deficiency become anaemic slowly, usually tolerate the low Hb levels remarkably well, and are rarely acutely confused at the time of presentation. However, B_{12} deficiency can result in a reversible chronic confusional state which can masquerade as dementia, though this is rare.

Brisk bleeding from any site will often result in a sufficient fall in cardiac output to compromise CNS function, with consequent confusion. Upper GI bleeding can go unnoticed and not infrequently presents as acute confusion in older patients.

Most patients with atrial fibrillation are not confused. Atrial fibrillation will only cause acute confusion when its sudden onset, with a rapid (>120/min) ventricular rate, results in heart failure and hypoxia.

Pneumonia often presents as confusion in elderly patients, particularly when hypoxia is present. However, old people with small patches of lung consolidation and without hypoxia can also be acutely confused, hence the need for careful physical examination of the chest and a chest radiograph in such patients.

Hypertension does not cause confusion unless complications such as heart failure, myocardial infarction, renal failure or stroke occur.

Question D

The results of the urgent initial investigations are normal. This is useful information insofar as it reinforces the contention that sensory deprivation, coupled with unfamiliar surroundings, was the reason for her acute confusion.

Question E

The first step in management is to replace her hearing aid battery, then at least an attempt can be made to talk to her. She should be repeatedly reassured, preferably by one nurse who should remain with her as much as possible during the episode. She should stay in the same position in the ward, to enable her to grasp the layout of her new surroundings. Sedation might be required initially, particularly if anxiety or hallucinations are a prominent feature; chlorpromazine or haloperidol are suitable, and often have to be given by intramuscular injection, in these circumstances.

Question F

Ideally the patient would return to her own home, where the familiar environment would help to keep her orientated; this would only have been possible if her husband had been well enough to look after her. A supply of hearing aid batteries would certainly be of value. After discharge, the patient's family doctor and relatives should be warned that changes of surroundings might lead to confusion.

Question G   4 is true.

More acutely confused elderly women than men are seen by physicians but this is because there are more elderly women than elderly men; the sexes appear to be equally susceptible. Formed delusions are a feature of psychoses, particularly paranoid schizophrenia and severe depression; the delusions of acute confusion are fleeting and ill-formed. The pressure of thought and speech which occur in mania are characteristic and usually easily distinguished from confusion. Occasionally severe acute mania presents as an apparent acute confusional state, though there is usually a history of manic depressive illness. Although a degree of bewilderment is often noticed in patients with a new stroke, most are not acutely confused. However, stroke can cause a florid acute confusional state, even when the abnormal neurological signs are relatively slight.

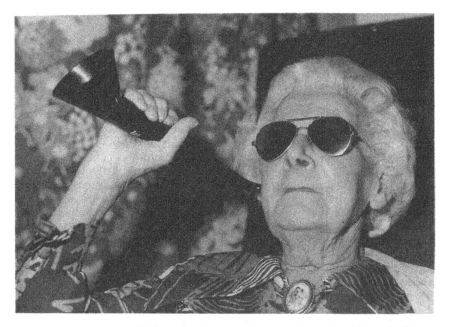

Figure 3 Sensory deprivation

It is always essential to consider drugs as the cause of acute confusion. However, stopping all medications reflexly is not wise, particularly if the patient is taking, for example, long-term cortico-steroids, oral antihyperglycaemic agents or insulin.

Suggested further reading

Hamilton C R Jr (1971) Giant cell arteritis: including temporal arteritis and poly-myalgia rheumatica. Medicine, 50, 1

Lipowski Z J (1983) Transient cognitive disorders (delirium, acute confusional states) in the elderly. American Journal of Psychiatry, 140, 1426-1436

Neshkes R E, Jarvik L F (1985) The central nervous system - dementia and delirium in old age. In: Brocklehurst J C (ed.) Textbook of Geriatric Medicine and Gerontology, 3rd Edn. Churchill Livingstone, Edinburgh

CASE 4

FALLS AND CONFUSION - 2

HISTORY

A lady of 70 presented to the outpatient clinic. She was super-
ficially lucid but unable to give a consistent history. Her daughter
said that the patient was quite well until about 6 weeks ago, since
when there had been a considerable decline in the patient's mobility
because of unsteadiness on her feet; two falls had occurred in the
previous week. Also over the past month, there had been increasing
forgetfulness and several episodes of confusion. The patient complained of frequent frontal headaches for the past month, these had
no particular diurnal pattern, though they occurred on most days,
lasted 2-3 hours, and were relieved by Distalgesic (paracetamol and
dextropropoxyphene). There was no history of a head injury
preceding the present illness. The patient had suffered a mild
chronic anxiety state for many years and this had been exacerbated
when her husband had a myocardial infarction 9 weeks ago. She was
taking Distalgesic, 2 as required and Librium (chlordiazepoxide),
5 mg daily.

Question A

Discuss:

What importance do you attach to this patient's complaint of
headache?

EXAMINATION

She was orientated in time, place and person. The chest, abdomen
and cardiovascular systems were normal; blood pressure
160/100 mmHg. The rectum was full of firm faeces. The cranial
nerves, pupils and optic fundi were normal. Tone was slightly increased in both limbs on the left; extension at the elbow was
slightly weak in the left arm, and movements of the left arm and leg
were slightly ataxic when tested formally. There was no detectable
asymmetry in the reflexes and the plantar responses were both
flexor. Her balance was very poor and the gait was ataxic. Sensory examination was normal.

Question B

True or false?

1. She has had a stroke, which accounts for all her symptoms
    and physical signs.

2. The presentation is in keeping with a diagnosis of multi-infarct dementia.

3. The minimal physical signs are unlikely to be of clinical relevance.

4. Normal pupils rule out an intracranial expanding lesion in this patient.

5. Normal pressure hydrocephalus is a possible diagnosis.

INVESTIGATIONS

Full blood count, blood urea, creatinine, glucose and electrolytes were all normal. Urine microscopy and culture were normal. Chest radiograph normal.

A computed tomography head scan was performed (Figure 4).

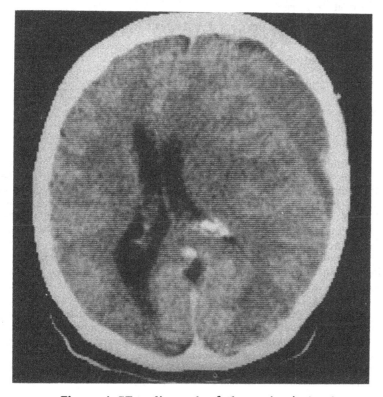

Figure 4 CT radiograph of the patient's head

Question C

Discuss:

What is the abnormality on this CT head scan?

Question D

Discuss:

1.   What is the treatment?

2.   When should rehabilitation begin?

Question E

True or false?

After evacuation of a subdural haematoma:

1.   A low serum sodium would suggest inappropriate ADH secretion.

2.   Six weeks antibiotic cover is needed, to avoid meningitis.

3.   The patient should not receive anticoagulant therapy at any time after surgery.

4.   Headache usually persists for several weeks.

5.   A follow-up CT head scan is unlikely to reveal clinically useful information.

ANSWERS

Question A

When the history of headache has spanned many years, it is unlikely to have a serious organic cause. However, frequent or persistent headache of recent onset such as this always needs to be considered carefully. The causes and patterns of headache in the elderly are much the same as those in younger individuals. This patient's complaint of several weeks of intermittent headache occurring at unpredictable times of the day or night, lasting up to 3 hours and being relieved by a mild analgesic should prompt investigation for intracranial pathology, particularly since there is also a history of intellectual and locomotor decline. The patient's history of chronic anxiety is misleading; it would be unwise to ascribe headache of this pattern to tension. In the elderly with headache it is particularly important to keep in mind temporal arteritis, depression, cervical spondylosis and intracranial haematoma as these are sometimes missed, with serious consequences. Paget's disease of the skull and unobvious stroke are causes of headache seen mainly in the elderly.

Question B   2 and 5 are true.

Stroke is certainly a possible explanation for the findings on physical examination, but the history is not that of stroke which usually has an abrupt onset with a tendency for improvement, rather than

20

progressive deterioration, to occur. Multi-infarct dementia can present with episodic confusion, focal neurological signs and declining mobility, though the history of headache would be unusual and the history in this case is rather too short for multi-infarct dementia.

Some of the most important physical signs are subtle; asymmetry of tone and reflexes are always of clinical importance and require explanation. In the context of headache and episodic confusion, all neurological signs should be considered to be of possible diagnostic value, particularly if they have recently emerged or changed.

Pupillary inequality is a relatively late sign of an expanding intracranial lesion and is probably due to pressure of the herniating temporal lobe on the oculomotor nerve, usually on the ipsilateral side. Consciousness is usually impaired before pupillary dilatation occurs in intracranial haematoma. On the other hand, elderly people often have pupils of unequal size, and though such pupils tend to be small and have preserved reaction to light, this can lead to diagnostic confusion.

Normal pressure hydrocephalus should be included in the differential diagnosis of a patient with these symptoms and signs, though the more usual presentation is of hypertonia, urinary incontinence and intellectual decline without headache or confusional episodes.

Question C

There is a large area of low attenuation between the skull vault and the right frontoparietal region with considerable shift of the ventricles and midline structures. These are the appearances of a fairly chronic subdural haematoma. When the haematoma is recent, the space-occupying lesion is more radio-opaque due to the presence of a large amount of blood, which is absorbed as time passes so that a very chronic haematoma will contain relatively radiolucent fluid. This example falls about midway between these extremes.

Question D

Neurosurgical referral for evacuation of the haematoma through burrholes is the treatment. The sooner the diagnosis is made, and the operation performed, the better the chances of neurosurgical improvement. Follow-up scans will detect any further build-up of fluid, in which case repeated evacuation through the existing burrholes might be needed. Passive physiotherapy should begin in the immediate post-operative period, and rehabilitation with the aim of restoring the maximum possible independence should begin as soon as the patient is ready to come off bed rest. Neurological recovery is sometimes excellent, in which case only a brief period of rehabilitation will be needed, as was the case with this patient.

21

Question E 1 is true.

Trauma, and probably surgery, to the head, is a cause of inappropriate ADH secretion, which can also occur in subdural haematoma. If inappropriate ADH secretion persists after evacuation of the clot, this may be due to incomplete removal of the haematoma, recurrence of the haematoma, post-operative intracerebral infection or other causes, for example a chest infection, unrelated to the haematoma.

Prolonged antibiotic cover is not necessary after surgery, though clinicians involved in the rehabilitation of a patient after discharge from the neurosurgical unit should be vigilant for the symptoms and signs of pyogenic meningitis.

A previous history of intracranial haematoma should not prevent the careful use of anticoagulants for the treatment of, for example, pulmonary embolism. Prolonged use of anticoagulants should be avoided if possible in such patients, particularly if there is a history of falls, alcohol abuse or CT scan evidence of cerebral atrophy.

The headache of intracranial haematoma is usually relieved promptly by clot evacuation; a cause should be sought if headache persists.

The main value of a follow-up CT head scan is in the detection of incomplete evacuation of the clot, recurrence of the clot and accumulation of encysted fluid, particularly after evacuation of chronic subdural haematomas. Decisions as to whether further surgical treatment is needed will largely depend on this investigation.

Suggested further reading

Markwallader T M (1981) Chronic subdural haematomas: a review. Journal of Neurosurgery, **54**, 637-645

Neshkes R E, Jarvik L F (1985) The central nervous system - dementia and delirium in old age. In: Brocklehurst J C (ed.) Textbook of Geriatric Medicine and Gerontology, 3rd Edn. Churchill Livingstone, Edinburgh

Pathy M S F (1985) The central nervous system - clinical presentation and management of neurological disorders in old age. In: Brocklehurst J C (ed.) Textbook of Geriatric Medicine and Gerontology, 3rd Edn. Churchill Livingstone, Edinburgh

CASE 5

ACUTE CONFUSION AND INCONTINENCE OF URINE

HISTORY

In July 1984, a 78-year-old lady, who lived alone, was found crawling about on the floor of her house by a neighbour, who called for an ambulance. A week earlier she had been very well, doing all her own shopping, housework and cooking. She had never been admitted to hospital before, though, according to her general practitioner, she had been treated by him with salbutamol tablets for "bronchitis" for about 3 years.

An interview with her daughter confirmed the medical history, and it was ascertained that the patient had probably taken no medication for several months and had never smoked.

Question A

True or false?

1.   Hypothermia can be ruled out because the weather was warm.

2.   Lower respiratory tract infections in old people occur less frequently in the summer months.

3.   The patient is likely to be dehydrated.

4.   The smoking history is probably irrelevant.

INITIAL EXAMINATION

She was disorientated in place and time, unkempt, and her clothes smelt of urine. Heart rate 124 per minute, blood pressure 130/80 mmHg, no signs of heart failure. High pitched expiratory rhonchi were noted throughout both lung fields. No definite focal neurological signs were found. The abdominal and rectal examinations were normal. The patient was unco-operative during the physical examination.

Question B

Since the patient is too confused to co-operate, which other signs of significant airflow obstruction should be looked for?

FURTHER EXAMINATION

The respiratory frequency was 32 per minute. It was thought that there was not cyanosis of the tongue and buccal mucous membranes, and the blood pressure was found to be 130/80 mmHg during expiration and 105/65 mmHg on inspiration.

Question C

In view of these findings would you:

1. Let the patient settle overnight and re-examine her the next day?

2. Sedate the patient and try to examine her more thoroughly?

3. Give intravenous normal saline to raise the blood pressure?

4. Consider the diagnosis of asthma?

5. Tell the patient's relatives that no treatment is likely to help and that the prognosis is poor?

Question D

Which investigations should be performed urgently?

1. A full blood count

2. Arterial blood gases

3. Chest radiograph

4. Blood urea and electrolytes

5. ECG

INVESTIGATIONS

PaO_2 51 mmHg (6.7 kPa) $PaCO_2$ 63 mmHg (8.1 kPa)   pH 7.40
The chest radiograph showed a small (10%) left pneumothorax.

Question E

As part of the management would you:

1. Pass a urinary catheter to control her incontinence?

2. Restrict oxygen supplementation to 28%?

3. Avoid the use of corticosteroid in a patient of this age?

4. Aspirate the pneumothorax?

5. Ventilate the patient if her $PaCO_2$ rises by 10 mmHg over the next 2 hours?

ANSWERS

Question A   2 and 3 are true.

Hypothermia occurs more frequently when ambient temperatures are low in winter; however, when individuals are rendered susceptible to hypothermia by abnormalities of thermoregulation, malnutrition, drugs (e.g. phenothiazines), hypothyroidism, dementia, alcoholism, trauma, haemorrhage or prolonged exposure, core temperature can fall despite a relatively warm ambient temperature.

Serious lower respiratory infection is seen throughout the year in elderly people in Britain, though admissions to hospital for pneumonia are much more frequent in the winter; preceding viral upper and lower respiratory tract infection probably predisposes the patient to secondary bacterial infection.

There is evidence that many elderly patients admitted to hospital in a confused state are dehydrated. This is probably more likely when admission is delayed, for example, when the patient lives alone, and when the ambient temperature is high.

The smoking history is important; the fact that the patient has never smoked throws considerable doubt on her diagnosis of "bronchitis", and should alert the physician to the possibility that other cardiac or respiratory pathology might be present.

Question B

The patient was already noted to have a tachycardia and expiratory rhonchi; it was important to count her respiratory frequency, look for central cyanosis, and observe for pulsus paradoxus when taking the blood pressure. A prolongation of the expiratory phase of the breath cycle is also worth looking for. These signs can usually be found even when the patient is confused. Such patients are unable to perform forced expiratory time, peak flow or vitalograph manoeuvres.

Question C   4 is correct.

The possibility of asthma should be considered in a patient of any age who is unwell and has physical signs of airflow obstruction. The combination of expiratory rhonchi, tachycardia and significant pulsus paradoxus is highly suggestive of asthma. It must be remembered that the confused elderly patient might not complain of breathlessness.

Leaving the patient to settle overnight under these circumstances is negligent. A vigorous approach to diagnosis is essential; untreated asthma is potentially fatal.

Sedation would be hazardous, the resulting fall in respiratory drive would lead to rapidly worsening hypoxia and hypercapnia particularly in a patient who is fatigued from prolonged airflow obstruction. Physical examination of confused patients should be done patiently and opportunistically, sometimes by returning to the patient on several occasions.

It makes no sense physiologically to give intravenous saline to such a patient. The relatively low blood pressure on inspiration during pulsus paradoxus probably results from impaired filling of the ventricles as the pericardium is stretched by the combination of diaphragmatic contraction and lung hyperinflation; severe acute left ventricular failure can be precipitated. If the patient is thought to be dehydrated an attempt should be made to give oral fluids or, failing that, intravenous 5% dextrose.

The relatives should be told that the illness is serious, but that investigations will be performed and treatment given accordingly.

Question D   2 and 3 are correct.

A chest radiograph must be performed as an emergency in an acutely confused patient with signs of intrathoracic pathology. When the signs are those of airflow obstruction, it is vital to rule out a pneumothorax, which might require aspiration. A pneumonia can also be obscured by the signs of airflow obstruction.

Despite the lack of clinical cyanosis, arterial blood gas tensions must be measured urgently, otherwise significant hypoxia might go undiagnosed and ventilatory failure, indicated by a rising CO_2 tension, will not be noticed until it is severe. Treatment cannot be properly planned unless the blood gases are known.

In the patient described there is no need to obtain a blood count, urea and electrolytes or ECG as an urgency, though they should be measured within a couple of days of admission.

Question E   4 and 5 are true.

When a patient is acutely confused and incontinent it is preferable to avoid a urinary catheter since the incontinence is likely to disappear once the cause of the confusion is treated. Urinary catheterisation always carries the risk of introducing infection into the bladder, no matter how carefully it is performed, and a small number of patients run the risk of Gram negative septicaemia when catheterised.

It is not necessary to restrict oxygen supplementation to 28% when patients have acute respiratory failure due to asthma; such patients usually maintain a good respiratory drive and do not depend on hypoxia to stimulate ventilation. Furthermore, elderly patients tolerate hypoxia poorly and should therefore be oxygenated vigorously.

Moderate to severe attacks of asthma in old age require corticosteroid treatment, and generally speaking, the doses used should be the same as those given to younger adults.

The occurrence of a pneumothorax during an attack of asthma can lead to a drastic worsening of the patient's condition; under these circumstances aspiration should be performed even when the pneumothorax appears to be quite small radiologically. This patient's

$PaCO_2$ was 61 mmHg, indicating moderately severe ventilatory failure, to which the pneumothorax would be contributing.

A marked rise in the $PaCO_2$ despite adequate treatment indicates worsening ventilatory failure, often because the asthmatic is fatigued, and artificial ventilation should be started. Age is not a bar to ventilation for the treatment of asthma.

Suggested further reading

Barr M L, Charles T J, Roy K, Seaton A (1979) Asthma in the elderly: an epidemiological survey. British Medical Journal, 1, 1041-1044

Liston E H (1982) Delirium in the aged. In: Jarvik L F and Small G W (eds.) The Psychiatric Clinics of North America, W B Saunders Co, Philadelphia

Neshkes R E, Jarvik L F (1985) The central nervous sytem - dementia and delirium in old age. In: Brocklehurst J C (ed.) Textbook of Geriatric Medicine and Gerontology, 3rd Edn. Churchill Livingstone, Edinburgh

CASE 6

MULTIPLE PATHOLOGY

HISTORY

A 75-year-old lady was admitted urgently with a 3-day history of worsening dyspnoea, anterior chest pain, and cough which was productive of a small volume of pale yellow sputum. Her ankles had been swollen for 3 weeks.

She had a history of exertional dyspnoea, orthopnoea and occasional paroxysmal nocturnal dyspnoea for many years. She had had rheumatic fever in childhood and had been told on several occasions that she had a heart murmur. She had had at least two proven myocardial infarctions. Her appetite was poor.

She lived alone and seldom got out of her flat; she neither smoked nor drank alcohol. Before admission her drugs comprised of choline theophyllinate, frusemide, digoxin, and salbutamol by tablet and inhaler.

ON EXAMINATION

She was fully conscious. The rectal temperature was 36.7°C. Pulse 110 irregular. Blood pressure 125/85 mmHg, the first heart sound was loud and there was a quiet apical mid-diastolic murmur and late systolic murmur. The respiratory rate was 28/minute and there were widespread inspiratory and expiratory rhonchi. The abdomen and CNS were normal. There was bilateral pitting oedema up to the knees and varicose veins were present.

Question A

Which statements are correct?

1.   People almost never survive to this age with rheumatic valve disease.

2.   This patient's yellow sputum is diagnostic of a respiratory infection.

3.   This patient is predisposed to respiratory infection.

4.   A 1-minute rectal temperature measurement is more reliable than a 5-minute axillary temperature measurement.

5.   This patient probably does not have digoxin toxicity.

Question B

Which of the following investigations is likely to provide information useful in the initial management of the patient?

1. Sputum microscopy and culture.

2. Vitalographic measurement of vital capacity and FEV1.

3. A chest radiograph.

4. An ECG.

5. An echocardiogram.

Question C

What other investigations would be worthwhile during the first 48 hours of the patient's admission? Discuss.

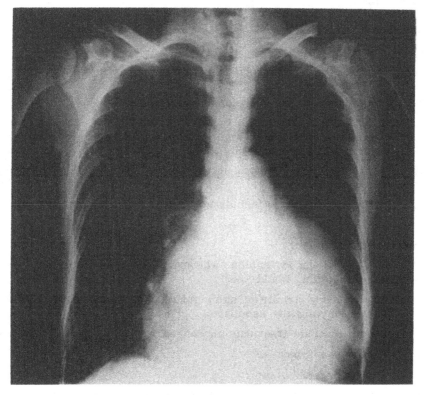

Figure 5 Chest radiograph

Question D

What are the abnormal features on the chest radiograph in Figure 5?

Question E

What is causing the patient's dyspnoea? Discuss.

Question F

Which of the following frequently have more than one cause in an individual old patient?

1. Dementia.

2. Ankle oedema.

3. Falls.

4. A Parkinsonian tremor.

5. Iron deficiency anaemia.

TREATMENT

Question G

Which is the optimal initial drug regimen in this patient?

1. Nebulised salbutamol/high dose steroid/oxygen/stop the other drugs.

2. Salbutamol inhaler/steroid inhaler/antibiotic/stop the other drugs.

3. Nebulised salbutamol/high dose steroid/oxygen/continue digoxin and frusemide only.

4. Intravenous salbutamol/intravenous aminophylline/oxygen/ continue digoxin only.

5. Nebulised salbutamol/nebulised steroid/stop the other drugs.

Question H

The patient developed angina whenever she was receiving her nebulised salbutamol. Would you:

1. Give glyceryl trinitrate sublingually or by transdermal patch before starting the nebuliser?

2. Simply continue treatment unchanged?

3. Prescribe a β-blocker?

4. Stop giving salbutamol?

5. Give glyceryl trinitrate sublingually or by transdermal patch and change from air to oxygen to drive the nebuliser?

ANSWERS

Question A   3, 4 and 5 are correct.

Survival into old age with rheumatic mitral valve disease is not rare, probably because of improved medical and surgical management earlier in life. Occasionally the diagnosis of mitral stenosis is established for the first time when the patient has reached old age. Patients with rheumatic aortic incompetence are only likely to live beyond middle age if prosthetic valve surgery is performed.

Yellowness of the sputum indicates the presence of leukocytes; this may be caused by infection or by other inflammatory conditions, of which asthma is the commonest (eosinophils usually predominate in asthmatic sputum).

Chronic respiratory disease of virtually any nature is associated with a predisposition to respiratory infection. Old age is in itself a risk factor for pneumonia. Patients with mitral valve disease, or with heart failure from any cause, have a higher incidence of lower respiratory tract infection.

Most clinical thermometers equilibrate within about 30 seconds. For practical purposes, rectal temperature is the same as core temperature, therefore a 1-minute reading will always accurately reflect core temperature. The temperature of tissue in the axilla takes up to 5 minutes to reach a plateau, and if the axilla is momentarily opened, a further 5 minutes is required. Therefore, there is much more likelihood of an erroneously low reading. Similarly, oral temperature takes about 3 minutes or more to become constant.

The only symptom she has which could be caused by digoxin toxicity is a poor appetite. Also, in atrial fibrillation the ventricular rate is usually much lower than 110 when the patient is digitalised at the therapeutic or toxic level. However, the only way to be certain is to measure the serum digoxin level (blood must be taken at least 6 hours after the last dose).

Question B   3 and 4

A chest radiograph is essential to assess the heart size and contour and to detect pulmonary oedema and pneumonia; the physical signs are often very unreliable in a patient such as this. An ECG will confirm the atrial fibrillation and in view of the anterior chest pain, might indicate a further myocardial infarction or ischaemia.

Question C

Sputum examination with H and E and Gram stains is worthwhile. If large numbers of intracellular pneumococci are seen, it is likely that any pneumonic shadowing on the radiograph is due to pneumococcal infection. Sputum culture is rarely useful, except when TB is suspected. If eosinophils predominate the diagnosis of asthma is likely, whereas neutrophils usually predominate in respiratory infection.

Arterial blood gases should be measured in all breathless patients, even if clinical cyanosis is not apparent. A full blood count should be performed and, if there is a leukocytosis, a differential white cell count done. Blood urea, glucose and electrolyte measurements are indicated in view of the patient's background history, and drug treatment. If the patient is able to perform a vitalograph manoeuvre, the FEV and FVC should be obtained; these can be repeated at a later date to ascertain whether reversible airflow obstruction occurred.

Blood cultures should be taken on all ill elderly patients with a cardiac murmur, even if the temperature and white blood cell count are normal, to rule out bacterial endocarditis.

An echocardiogram will often give a useful assessment of the mitral valve and can sometimes detect the presence of vegetations caused by bacterial endocarditis.

Asymptomatic urinary infection is so common, particularly in elderly women, that a routine MSSU for microscopy and culture should be collected from all patients admitted to the geriatric wards.

The patient gave a history of anterior chest pain and is known to have had previous myocardial infarctions, therefore cardiac enzyme concentrations should be measured to detect further myocardial necrosis.

Question D

The chest radiograph shows a cardiac contour typical of severe left atrial enlargement secondary to mitral valve disease. The lung fields are markedly hyperinflated with low flat hemidiaphragms.

Question E

This is an example of how multiple pathology can result in diagnostic difficulties by causing one predominant symptom; the patient's dyspnoea is partly due to airflow obstruction and partly to mitral valve disease. The long history of exertional dyspnoea and orthopnoea was almost certainly due to mitral stenosis. However, her airflow obstruction was of fairly recent onset and she had never smoked, which makes asthma the most likely additional diagnosis. Treatment should be based on the assumption that the airflow obstruction is likely to be reversible; furthermore, the chest radiograph does not show pulmonary oedema, so it is probable that when the patient was at rest in the sitting position, the mitral valve disease was not causing the major component of her dyspnoea.

Question F

Dementia, Parkinsonian tremors and iron deficiency are usually, though not invariably, caused by a single disease process in any individual, for example, Alzheimer's disease, phenothiazines and carcinoma of the caecum, respectively.

On the other hand, ankle oedema is often the result of a number of physiological abnormalities in a given patient: right heart failure, dependent posture (e.g. sleeping in a chair), hypoproteinaemia, incompetent leg vein valves, bilateral deep venous thrombosis, drug induced salt and water retention, poor use of the calf muscle "pump" - these may occur singly but are frequently present in combinations of two or more. Treatment needs to be directed at all the contributing factors if it is to be successful.

Similarly, falls are often the consequence of an accumulation of factors which interfere with postural control; for example, a patient with Parkinson's disease might not start falling until a hypnotic is prescribed, or a patient with poor sight caused by diabetic retinopathy does not fall despite her co-existent painful osteoarthrotic left hip until she develops a peripheral sensory neuropathy and becomes uncertain of her footing.

Other important examples are acute confusion, urinary incontinence and easy fatiguability.

Question G 3

Regimens 2, 4 and 5 do not include adequate steroid therapy, which is an essential part of the treatment of asthma of this severity. Regimens 2 and 5 omit oxygen, which should be given despite the fact that the patient's PaO_2 is not very low. Antibiotics are not indicated as there is no convincing clinical or radiological evidence of a bacterial respiratory infection; furthermore, a blood culture series to rule out SABE is more reliable when antibiotics are not being administered. It is sensible to continue the patient's customary doses of digoxin and frusemide initially, as these appear to have been adequately controlling her cardiac condition prior to the relapse of her asthma and there is no good reason to consider that she was either over-digitalised or volume depleted. Salbutamol is most effectively given by jet nebulisation in severe asthma; metered dose inhalers are not easy to use when the patient is very breathless, and salbutamol and choline theophyllinate tablets are of little value in asthma in relapse.

Question H 5

The patient has valvular heart disease and is at considerable risk of developing severe heart failure if the myocardium becomes hypoxic; angina is a symptom of myocardial hypoxia, and should prompt immediate treatment in these circumstances. The asthma must be treated adequately, which excludes option 4. A β-blocker could worsen the asthma and might precipitate left ventricular failure.

Nitrates effectively relieve angina in these circumstances, but will do so more easily if the patient is well oxygenated, so option 5 is preferable to option 1. It must be remembered that patients with chronic CO_2 retention might severely underventilate if given such high concentrations of oxygen to breathe. Also, most jet nebulisers require a driving gas flow rate of 6-8 litres/minute, which can be achieved with standard oxygen valves used in hospitals, though the oxygen valves fitted to portable oxygen cylinders often give a maximum flow rate of only 4 litres/minute, which might not adequately nebulise the drug solution.

Suggested further reading

Caird F I, Dall J L C, Kennedy R D (eds.) (1976) Cardiology in Old Age, Plenum Press, New York

Clark T J H, Godfrey S (eds.) (1983) Asthma, Chapman and Hall, London

Pomerance A (1981) Cardiac pathology in the elderly. In: Noble R J and Rothbaum D A (eds.) Geriatric Cardiology, F A Davies Co, Philadelphia

CASE 7

FALLS AND DIARRHOEA

HISTORY

A general practitioner telephones you to ask your advice on the management of Mr J N, a 77-year-old widower who has had diarrhoea for 4 days and has fallen twice in the past 24 hours. The GP says he saw the patient 2 weeks ago and treated him for a chest infection; until then the patient had been in good health and had rarely visited the general practitioner. He smoked a pipe. Now, the patient has a heart rate of 105/minute and a supine blood pressure of 110/65 mmHg.

Question A

What other information would you ask the GP for at this stage? Discuss.

Question B

The patient lives alone. Would you:

1. Arrange an immediate admission to hospital for assessment and treatment?

2. Do a domiciliary assessment visit the following evening?

3. Advise the GP to give symptomatic treatment and let you know if the patient does not improve?

4. List the patient for an out-patient consultation?

5. Suggest that the diarrhoea be treated symptomatically and arrange for the patient to attend your Day Hospital for falls recovery practice?

ON EXAMINATION

He was fully conscious and orientated. His tissue turgor seemed low and his tongue was dry and coated. Pulse 112/minute. Blood pressure 120/70 mmHg lying, 105/60 mmHg sitting; there was some tenderness on deep palpation of the left iliac fossa, the rectum was empty and normal. His left arm was freshly bruised over the lateral aspect of the elbow. Rectal temperature 36.8°C.

He vomited during the physical examination. Prior to his acute illness he had been taking ampicillin (prescribed for the recent chest infection) and Senokot every other night for several years.

35

Question C

True or false?

1. Low tissue turgor is a reliable guide to the presence of dehydration in this patient.

2. Grey-brown coating of the dorsum of the tongue is usually caused by dehydration.

3. Antibiotic hypersensitivity was the likely mechanism of his low sitting blood pressure.

4. Postural hypotension is a frequent sign of salt and water depletion in old people.

5. His diarrhoea was probably caused by laxative abuse.

Question D

Which of the following investigations will give information useful in the immediate management of the patient?

1. ESR

2. Haematocrit

3. Blood urea and electrolytes

4. Stool culture

5. Plain abdominal radiograph

Question E

By what method would you replace the patient's fluid and how would you assess the patient's state of hydration during the first few days of treatment?

The patient was given no drugs and his state of hydration, as judged clinically and by laboratory investigations, improved. However, 6 days after admission he still complained of having four or five loose stools per day with tenesmus.

Question F

Would you:

1. Reassure the patient that his diarrhoea would soon settle spontaneously, and discharge him home?

2. Examine the stool for the presence of parasites?

3. Give loperamide (Imodium) and discharge him once his diarrhoea stopped?

4. Test the stool and blood for the presence of Clostridium difficile toxin?

5. Measure the faecal fat content?

INVESTIGATIONS

The test for <u>Clostridium difficile</u> toxin was positive.

Question G

The next stage in management is:

1. Continue to maintain hydration and allow the pseudo-membranous colitis to settle.

2. Oral metronidazole.

3. Intravenous vancomycin.

4. Parenteral penicillin and gentamicin.

5. Oral vancomycin.

Question H

What cautionary note should be included in the patient's discharge letter to the GP?

ANSWERS

Question A

It is important to know whether the patient lives alone or with a competent relative, as this will determine to a large extent whether the patient is looked after at home or in hospital. Details of the patient's drug history should be enquired about, particularly whether or not new treatment has been started recently, and what was prescribed for the chest infection. The GP will probably know whether the patient is willing to be admitted to hospital immediately if that is thought necessary. The GP might know whether the patient's usual supine blood pressure is higher than 110/65 mmHg.

Question B   1

Immediate admission is the best course of action in this case because the patient lives alone, has been falling and has signs of volume depletion, probably as a result of his diarrhoea. Domiciliary assessment within a few hours would be reasonable, but would probably result in admission to hospital anyway; to leave the patient for more than 24 hours without assessment would be negligent. Symptomatic treatment with, for example, Lomotil, and oral rehydration could only be properly performed if the patient has an able-bodied attendant. Clinic assessment would result in too long a delay. Falls recovery practice is appropriate for patients who habitually fall and in whom the cause of the falls is not easily treated; this does not apply to this patient, who may well stop falling once his acute illness is treated.

Mr J N was admitted to the acute assessment ward.

Question C   4 is true.

Tissue turgor is not a good guide to the state of hydration in old people, in whom the skin and subcutaneous tissues are lax as the result of ageing changes and, sometimes, weight loss.

Many factors influence the state of the tongue; the grey-brown coating seen in this patient could be associated with the recent upper respiratory infection, antibiotic treatment or pipe smoking.

Antibiotic hypersensitivity could cause postural hypotension, though in this case the salt and water depletion caused by diarrhoea is the most likely reason. Most elderly patients with salt and water depletion have a significant fall in blood pressure in the erect position; this usually responds to fluid replacement.

Laxative abuse is a cause of diarrhoea; however, as this patient has been using Senokot in moderate amounts for many years, it is unlikely to be the cause of his recent illness.

Question D   2 and 3

When the circulating blood volume is reduced by dehydration, the haematocrit is raised proportionally; this is of particular use if the patient's usual haematocrit is known (which is often the case when patients are well known to geriatric units) and for comparison after fluid replacement has been given. The blood urea is usually raised when dehydration is moderate to severe; haemoconcentration and a low renal blood flow are the most likely mechanisms. If the patient's renal function is essentially normal, the blood creatinine concentration will be normal or only slightly elevated in these circumstances. In true dehydration (e.g. when the patient is not drinking), the serum sodium is usually elevated, whereas in the salt and water depletion of prolonged vomiting and diarrhoea, the serum sodium is usually within the normal range, or, if the patient has been drinking water, it may be low. After prolonged sweating, with access to water but inadequate salt replacement, the sodium is usually low. Thus, measurement of the blood urea and electrolytes as an urgency allows a rational approach to fluid replacement to be made.

The ESR is of no immediate use in a patient with an acute diarrhoeal illness; though of course it can be elevated in conditions such as ulcerative colitis.

Stool culture should be performed, but not as an urgency in this case, as it will not contribute to the immediate management. A plain abdominal radiograph is not required.

Question E

The patient has vomited, therefore, in view of his probable severe salt and water depletion, an intravenous infusion of normal saline is best. Potassium is lost in diarrhoea, and should be added to the infusion. In the absence of vomiting, particularly when the patient is not very ill, fluid replacement can be given orally in the form of a balanced salt solution (e.g. Dextrolyte or Rehidrat); this is also very useful for the management of milder cases in the patient's home. The aim should be to replace the patient's fluid over the 24 hours or so after admission. It is helpful to weigh the patient upon admission; a gain of at least 2-3 kg should occur over the first day of treatment. Urine volume should be measured; in a patient with normal renal function the urine output will begin to rise once fluid replacement is adequate. If the patient continues to produce less than 30 ml/hour it is likely that more fluid is required. The urine specific gravity will also fall once rehydration has been achieved. The haematocrit and blood urea should fall. The postural hypotension will improve, but may persist for a few days after fluid replacement is complete. If fluid is being given intravenously, a careful watch must be kept for signs of fluid overload, particularly breathlessness, an increase in respiratory rate, basal lung crepitations and a raised jugular venous pressure.

Question F   2 and 4

Stool culture will have been performed within the first day or so, though it might be helpful to repeat the culture at this stage. Several separate stool specimens should be examined for the presence of parasites. Pseudomembranous colitis, associated with the presence of Clostridium difficile is a known complication of oral antibiotic treatment, and it can present as an acute diarrhoeal illness. Stool and blood should be tested for Cl. difficile toxin, and the organism can also be cultured from stool. However, the organism can be present in the stool samples of individuals with no symptoms, or in patients with diarrhoea due to other causes; the detection of the toxin is therefore a more reliable guide to pseudomembranous colitis.

Suppression of the diarrhoea without an adequate diagnosis is not good policy. Though a specific diagnosis is often not made in acute diarrhoea, the patient should be observed carefully in hospital, or at home if the domestic support is adequate, investigated appropriately and seen by the physician or GP at least once for a follow-up assessment.

Steatorrhoea is rarely acute and not usually associated with tenesmus; faecal fat measurement is inconvenient for the patient and would not be likely to provide useful information in this case.

The clinician should examine the patient's stool, with particular attention to the presence of blood, pus, mucus and undigested food particles.

Question G   5

Oral vancomycin is the treatment for antibiotic-associated pseudomembranous colitis, though metronidazole has been used also; the other antibiotic regimens will either be ineffective, or could lead to worsening of the condition. Hydration should be maintained.

Question H

The GP should be informed that a spontaneous relapse of the pseudomembranous colitis might occur, and would require immediate readmission to hospital.

Suggested further reading

Bartlett J C (1978) Antibiotic-associated pseudomembranous colitis due to toxin-producing clostridia. New England Journal of Medicine, 298, 531

Lye M D W (1985) The melieu interieur and aging. In: Brocklehurst J C (ed.) Textbook of Geriatric Medicine and Gerontology, 3rd Edn. Churchill Livingstone, Edinburgh

CASE 8

DOMICILIARY VISIT
– ANKLE OEDEMA

HISTORY

A financially secure bachelor of 75 years of age was seen at home by a geriatrician at the request of the general practitioner. The patient was complaining of fluid oozing from the skin of both legs below the knees. He had suffered from chronic ankle swelling for at least 10 years. He lived alone and said that friends brought him whatever food he wanted. He had been taking frusemide, 40 mg daily for several years, though he was sceptical as to whether this had helped his swollen legs. The home was in a good state of repair, though untidy. The patient's bed was upstairs and he stated that he usually managed to get upstairs to sleep.

Question A

What other information should be sought during this domiciliary consultation? Discuss.

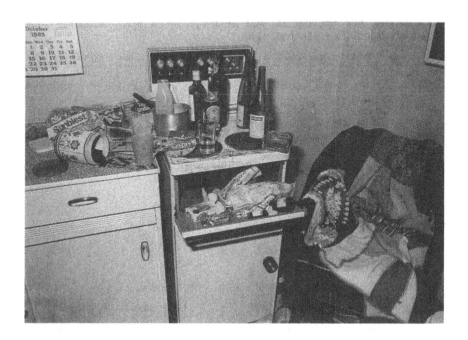

Figure 6 Reconstruction of the patient's kitchen/living room

Question B

Figure 6 is a reconstruction of the patient's kitchen/living room. What do you see that is of relevance to the case?

PHYSICAL EXAMINATION

He was unwilling to lie flat, so an examination was performed while he sat in a chair. He was fully orientated. There were Dupuytren's contractures of both hands. No abnormalities were detected in the chest, abdomen, heart or CNS. Both legs were swollen below the knees, the left more than the right; the left leg was redder and warmer than the right and had several pink/yellow superficial ulcers over the anterior and lateral aspects of the lower third which were exuding a clear fluid. There were no pressure sores and no sacral oedema.

Question C

Based on what you know of the patient, would you:

1. Increase the dose of frusemide, add spironolactone and ask the district nurse to dress the ulcers?

2. Admit him to hospital for further assessment and treatment?

3. Suggest that he admit himself to a nursing home?

4. Advise him to rest in bed at home for a week with his feet elevated, then see him again?

5. Refer him to the plastic surgeons for skin grafting of the leg ulcers?

After admission to hospital, a further physical examination, including a rectal examination, added no new information, though on the second day his axillary temperature was 37.9°C.

The results of screening investigations were as follows:

Haemoglobin 13.0 g/dl

White cell count 6.1×10^9/l (normal differential)

MCH   28 pg (normal 27-32)

MCHC   32.0 g/dl (normal 31-35)

MCV   104 fl (normal 80-97)

The blood film was normochromic with anisocytosis.

Na	139 mmol/l (132-144)	Ca	1.90 mmol/l (2.10-2.65)
K	4.4 mmol/l (3.5-5.0)	Phosphate	0.9 mmol/l (0.7-1.4)
Urea	4.1 mmol/l (2.5-7.5)	Glucose	8.5 mmol/l (3.2.-9.2)

Creatinine	0.09 mmol/l (0.01-0.12)		Total prot. 53 g/l (60-80)
			Albumin 24 g/l (33-38)
LDH	550 iu/l	(200-450)	MSSU - normal
ALT	11 iu/l	(5-40)	ECG - normal
GGT	92 iu/l	(5-65)	

Chest radiograph - slightly enlarged cardiac shadow, otherwise normal.

Urine sugar - negative

Urine protein - trace

Question D

From what you have learned about the patient, which of the following investigations should be done immediately?

1. Blood culture.

2. Plasma protein electrophoresis.

3. Another white blood cell count.

4. Swabs from the leg ulcers for bacterial culture.

5. Serum parathormone assays.

Question E

Explain the low serum calcium.

Question F

Name five other causes of ulceration of the skin below the knees which are common in older people.

After admission the patient was encouraged to remain mobile, he slept in a bed and elevated his legs while sitting. The dose of frusemide was kept at 40 mg daily, he was discouraged from adding salt to his food at the table and he was given protein supplements. The cellulitis was treated with oral erythromycin and cleared quickly.

His oedema rapidly improved, and his body weight fell by 6 kg over the first 2 weeks. The leg ulcers healed. His lying and standing blood pressures were satisfactory.

Three days after admission he became slightly disorientated, agitated and fidgety. There were no changes on physical examination, no fever and no substantial changes in his serum biochemistry or blood count; these symptoms resolved spontaneously after about 4 days.

Question G

His confusional state was probably due to which of the following?

1. Bacteraemia
2. Over-diuresis and volume depletion
3. Alcohol withdrawal
4. A change of environment
5. Erythromycin hypersensitivity

Question H

Taking into account the history, his lifestyle, physical findings, the results of investigations and the response to treatment, which of the following do you think contributed to his severe oedema?

1. Congestive heart failure
2. The nephrotic syndrome
3. Alcohol abuse
4. An inadequate diet
5. Sleeping in a chair

The patient said he would give up alcohol completely, he was discharged and remained well. Two months later all the biochemical and haematological indices were normal except the MCV which had risen to 114 fl.

Question I

Would you:

1. Take this to be evidence of continued drinking, advise him to stop, and repeat the test after a month?
2. Measure his serum B_{12} and folate levels?
3. Measure nothing, give an oral folic acid supplement and repeat the MCV after a month?
4. Arrange for a bone marrow examination?
5. Measure his leukocyte ascorbic acid levels?

Question J

What arrangements would you make to follow up this man after his discharge from the out-patient clinic?

ANSWERS

Question A

While still in the patient's house, specific enquiry should be made about how often the patient is unable to get upstairs, whether there is a stair rail and what prevents him from managing the stairs on certain days. Where does he sleep when he cannot manage to reach his bed? Have there been any falls? Is there a toilet downstairs? Is he incontinent? What heating is in the house? Who comes to help with his household chores? What does he eat exactly? Does anyone attend to his legs? Does he take his medication regularly?

The aim should be to try to build up a picture of how the patient is living; this often gives considerable insight into the patient's illness. A "birdseye view" of the patient's way of life is sometimes more useful than close scrutiny of one aspect of the physical examination or history when it comes to planning management. These impressions are often at their most vivid at the time of the initial domiciliary assessment.

Question B

Firstly, it is apparent that he rarely uses his cooker other than as a table top, suggesting that he might not be taking an adequate diet. The empty and half-empty spirit, wine and beer bottles indicate that his alcohol comsumption is probably high. There is evidence of cigarette smoking. His bottles of tablets are scattered about on the grill shelf; this could indicate that he is not careful about his medication. The chair looks as though it is used for sleeping in, not just for sitting. The kitchen is generally cluttered and untidy, so perhaps the patient has not been looking after himself very well.

Question C   2

Hospital admission for assessment is the best option in this case for the following reasons:

(a)   The cause, or causes, of his oedema are not known, and require investigation.

(b)   The recent worsening of the oedema and ulceration of the legs also require investigation and vigorous treatment.

(c)   He lives alone.

Increasing the diuretic dose would be only to treat the oedema "blind"; furthermore, it is unlikely to improve matters in a patient with oedema in the absence of signs of heart failure when a patient often sleeps in a chair with his legs down. The district nurse could dress the ulcers, though they are unlikely to heal until the oedema is reduced. If he rests in bed his oedema might settle, though again, this will not lead to a proper diagnosis and since he lives alone, he would find it virtually impossible to keep to bed rest. Also, it is generally not good policy to advise bed rest in elderly patients with poor mobility in view of the enhanced risks of venous thrombosis, pulmonary embolism, pressure sores and pneumonia, and postural hypotension on eventual rising from bed. Skin grafting would be of no use while severe oedema is present.

Question D   1 and 3

The patient has ulcers, a reddened left leg and has had a spike of fever; under these circumstances, it is likely that there is cellulitis complicating the oedema, and the offending organism will sometimes be isolated in blood. If the white cell count, particularly the neutrophil count, has risen this would support the contention that infection is present. If swabs from the ulcers are cultured there will almost always be organisms grown, though it is rarely possible to be certain that the same bacteria are causing the cellulitis; hence ulcer swabs are too misleading to be of value in planning antibiotic treatment.

Plasma protein electrophoresis would only confirm the hypoproteinaemic state and would add nothing to the diagnosis.

Parathormone assays are not indicated; the reasons are outlined in the answer to Question E.

Question E

The serum calcium is lowered in proportion to the low serum albumin, to which the larger proportion of the total calcium is bound. The ionised calcium will be normal, so there will be no symptoms or signs of hypocalcaemia, and the mechanisms controlling calcium homeostasis will be intact.

Question F

Ischaemic ulcers in patients with peripheral arteriosclerosis

Chronic varicose ulcers

Pressure sores

Ulcers caused by ill-fitting shoes

Trophic ulcers associated with peripheral sensory neuropathy (especially in diabetics)

Question G   3

The evidence for alcohol abuse was quite subtle in this case, but when all the pointers were considered together, it became much clearer. Despite the patient's protestations that he only had "a small sherry on Sundays and at Christmas", there were several sherry bottles and beer cans visible in his kitchen. There were no neurological or skeletomuscular abnormalities which would have prevented him from climbing his stairs; it was likely, therefore, that he was often too drunk to cope with them and so slept in the chair in his kitchen. He had a mild alcohol withdrawal syndrome, this is probably much more common than frank delirium tremens in elderly alcoholics. The raised GGT and LDH and low serum albumin are consistent with a high alcohol intake and low protein diet, and a raised MCV is a frequent finding. The absence of other obvious explanations for his condition should raise the question of alcohol abuse, and the rapid improvement when alcohol was stopped and a good diet given also supports the diagnosis. Severe craving for alcohol after admission to hospital is not often observed in elderly heavy drinkers.

His cellulitis was being treated, successfully, with erythromycin and he was neither febrile nor had he a leukocytosis, therefore bacteraemia or septicaemia is unlikely.

His diuretic dose had not been increased, and his fall in body weight was largely due to the shedding of oedema fluid once he started to sleep in bed. He had no other signs of hypovolaemia, such as postural hypotension.

Confusional states brought on by a change of environment usually occur at the time of admission, or during the first night after admission. Confusion due to antibiotic hypersensitivity would be accompanied by other signs of an antibiotic reaction such as pyrexia, hypotension, a rash or vomiting.

Question H   3, 4 and 5

This man's oedema is an example of a condition with multiple pathogeneses, in this case hypoproteinaemia, probably of dietary or hepatic origin, sleeping with his legs down, and possibly salt and water retention secondary to hepatic dysfunction, but with a single aetiology, alcohol abuse.

There were no physical signs or findings on investigation to warrant the diagnosis of congestive heart failure, and in the nephrotic syndrome there is always substantial proteinuria.

Question I   2

Since his other biochemical indices had returned to normal and he was looking and feeling well, it was unlikely that he had continued to abuse alcohol. Also, the MCV does not usually rise as high as 114 fl due to alcohol abuse alone. It would be prudent to measure his serum B_{12} and folate levels, though neither B_{12} nor folate supplements should be given until the results are known. If the B_{12} (as was the case in this man) or folate levels are low, it is not essential to examine the bone marrow. The MCV has been observed to be slightly raised in some patients with scurvy; however, there were no clinical indications to justify measurement of ascorbic acid levels in this patient.

47

Question J

The patient returned to his solitary lifestyle. Out-patient follow-up during the period immediately after discharge would allow a thorough review of his physical condition and gives an opportunity to reinforce the ban on alcohol; blood alcohol levels and appropriate biochemical indices could be measured. If he remains well and is discharged from the clinic, it would be advisable to arrange for a health visitor or district nurse to call on him from time to time, mainly to examine his legs and to try to ascertain whether he has returned to the bottle. An occasional visit by the general practitioner could achieve the same.

If the patient is willing to accept it, regular attendance at a luncheon club for the elderly would help to ensure a reasonable diet and provide some social life, both of which might reduce the likelihood of his lapsing back into alcohol abuse. Other arrangements will depend on the patient's tastes and interests, family support and on the types of amenities available.

Suggested further reading

Kass L (1976) Pernicious anaemia. In: Major Problems in Internal Medicine, Vol II. Saunders, Philadelphia

Mishara B L, Kasterbaum R (1980) Alcohol and Old Age. Grune and Stratton, New York

CASE 9

DIZZINESS

HISTORY

A lady of 85 years was admitted to hospital at the request of her general practitioner who was concerned by the patient's frequent complaints of "dizziness". That day she had had a fall which occurred as she was rising from the chair where she had been sleeping. She was not injured and was able to get up immediately. She also suffered from frontal headaches; these had been present on and off throughout adult life. Her "dizziness" was not related to posture, neck movements, the time of day, or to other symptoms. She described the "dizziness" as "everything just leaves me" or "I feel as though I'm going to pass out" or "my vision doesn't seem right". Sometimes the "dizziness" persisted throughout the day. However, she could not be more specific than this.

She lived with a man friend who gave her a lot of support and had recently been doing most of the domestic work. Her husband died 11 years ago. She had had no serious illnesses and was taking no drugs.

Question A

True or false?

Vertigo:

1. is often accompanied by horizontal nystagmus

2. is rarely associated with vomiting

3. is most often due to an anxiety state in old age

4. causes falls

5. can be a feature of vestibular neuronitis

Question B

True or false?

Vertigo in older adults

1. can be caused by vertebrobasilar insufficiency

2. is frequently caused by hypnotic drugs

3. is accompanied by deafness but not tinnitus in Ménière's disease

4. tests of vestibular function are usually normal

5. can be caused by chronic otitis media

EXAMINATION

She was thin (and said she always had been), fully orientated and anxious; she constantly fiddled with her clothes and bedsheets and had a fine tremor.

Question C

List the particular aspects of the physical examination that you would pay attention to in an old person complaining of "dizziness".

EXAMINATION AND INVESTIGATION

There were no other abnormalities on a full physical examination. The blood pressure was 160/105 mmHg lying and standing. A full blood count, ESR, routine biochemical profile, chest radiograph, and standard 12-lead ECG were all normal.

Question D

Discuss the relationship between this patient's "dizziness" and her recent falls.

Question E

Her "dizziness" was probably caused by which of the following?

1. Anxiety

2. Old age

3. Vertebrobasilar insufficiency

4. An intracranial space-occupying lesion

5. Hypertension

Question F

From what you know of the patient, which of the following investigations would you perform?

1. A 24-hour ambulatory ECG

2. T3, T4 and TSH assay

3. A radiograph of the cervical spine

4. A CT head scan

5. Aortic arch angiography

The patient had no falls after admission, though she complained of virtually constant "dizziness". She could not relax and slept badly. Her thyroid hormone assays were normal.

Question G

Would you:

1. Prescribe diazepam and discharge her?

2. Arrange a transfer to a psychiatric ward as soon as possible?

3. Interview the man she lives with to obtain more information about the patient?

4. Discharge her and arrange an out-patient appointment with a psychiatrist?

5. Prescribe an hypnotic and review her in your general out-patient clinic?

You find out that she has been anxious, fidgety and lacking in confidence for about 6 months; before that she was an outgoing lady though a little rigid in her ways.

Question H

Which of the following is the most likely diagnosis?

1. A late bereavement reaction

2. A chronic anxiety state

3. An agitated depression

4. Hypomania

5. Early dementia

Question I

How would you deal with this?

Nine months later she was feeling well; her friend confirmed that she was now her "old self". However, she had noticed a progressive decline in the "sharpness" of her vision.

Question J

Which of the following could cause this symptom?

1. Glaucoma

2. Senile macular degeneration

3. Cataract

4. A refractive error

5. Proliferative diabetic retinopathy

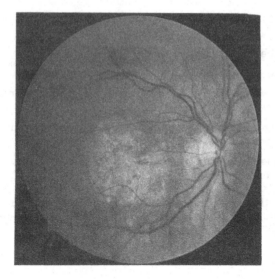

Figure 7 Retinal photograph

Question K

What is the diagnosis?

ANSWERS

Question A   1, 4 and 5 are true.

Vertigo results from disease of the eighth cranial nerve, including the labyrinth. In true vertigo the patient experiences a sensation of rotation of himself or his surroundings. Most "dizzy" old people do not have vertigo, and it is important to distinguish true vertigo from other forms of dizziness; true vertigo is almost always accompanied by nystagmus. Vomiting is common, particularly when the vertigo is acute in onset and severe. Anxiety states do not cause vertigo, though patients with vertigo are often very anxious. Old people find it virtually impossible to stand when they have vertigo, and an attack which begins while the person is ambulant can lead to a fall. Vertigo is often a feature of vestibular neuronitis; this condition probably occurs at all ages and is often preceded by a febrile illness such as a viral upper respiratory tract infection.

Question B   1 and 5 are true.

Vascular insufficiency of the vestibular system and its connections is probably one of the more common causes of vertigo in old age; degenerative disease of the vertebrobasilar arteries is the most likely reason in most cases. Brain stem strokes involving the eighth nerve also occur.

Tests of vestibular function, such as head tilting and caloric stimulation are usually abnormal in patients with vertigo.

The vertigo of Ménière's disease is usually episodic and accompanied by a gradual decline in hearing and worsening tinnitus. Very similar symptoms can be caused by chronic otitis media, which can occur at any age, and it is important to examine the tympanic membranes to differentiate these, since chronic otitis media is treatable.

The dizziness frequently experienced by patients taking psychotropic medication is not vertigo.

Question C

A full physical examination is needed, though the following deserve special attention:

Gait

Pulse

Blood pressure - lying and standing

Aortic valve - ? stenosis or incompetence

Carotid arteries - for bruits

Neck movements

Nystagmus

Hearing

Tympanic membranes

Gait If a patient claims to be "dizzy" and yet at the same time can walk safely with a normal gait, it is unlikely that he or she has vertigo, postural hypotension, cerebellar disease or "dizziness" of cardiac origin. Of course the gait may be normal between attacks of, for instance, Ménière's vertigo. Patients who walk about feeling "dizzy all the time" rarely have a physical illness.

Pulse The pulse may be slow, as in complete heart block or digitalis intoxication, or rapid, as in a supraventricular tachycardia, in which case the cause of the symptoms might be obvious. More often, the pulse will be normal, or that of a common arrhythmia, such as atrial fibrillation, and further investigation will be required to detect more subtle abnormalities of cardiac rhythm, for example, the sick sinus syndrome which can cause episodes of faintness, Stokes-Adams attacks or sudden death.

Blood pressure It is vital to measure the blood pressure with the patient lying and 2 minutes after standing to detect postural hypotension. A fall of systolic blood pressure of 20 mmHg upon standing is often accompanied by a feeling of faintness in old people, and lesser falls in standing blood pressure probably cause symptoms in some individuals.

Aortic valve Both aortic stenosis and incompetence can cause faintness due to a fall in cerebral blood flow. However, it must be remembered that aortic ejection systolic murmurs are common in old age and most are of little or no haemodynamic importance.

Carotid arteries Occasionally, patients with transient ischaemic attacks present with the complaint of "dizziness" though the majority present with transient unilateral weakness, paraesthesiae or amaurosis fugax. Some of these will have a carotid bruit.

Neck movements Rotation and extension of the neck may precipitate the symptoms of vertebrobasilar insufficiency, or vertigo due to inner ear disease; these can sometimes be illicited during the physical examination. Severely limited or painful neck movements can be caused by degenerative disease of the cervical vertebrae, which may be associated with vertebrobasiliar insufficiency.

Nystagmus is usually present or can be provoked in patients with vertigo and is a reliable sign of vestibular disease in patients complaining of a sense of rotation.

Hearing Hearing loss may be a feature of Ménière's disease, chronic otitis media, and drug ototoxicity, all of which may cause vertigo. Care must be taken not to confuse these with hearing loss due to wax in the external auditory meatus or presbyacusis; these do not cause "dizziness".

Tympanic membranes Auriscope examination should always be included in the examination of elderly patients as it will detect wax in the external auditory meatus, and enables acute and chronic otitis media, otitis externa and tympanic membrane perforation to be diagnosed.

Question D

The patient's "dizziness" was often present for many hours, was not vertigo or faintness and was associated with the fear of falling or passing out, though these events did not actually occur. She was able to quickly get up from the floor after her fall, which makes it unlikely to have been a drop attack. The fall could have been caused by postural hypotension, though this is unlikely as there was no reported faintness, she had no other symptoms of postural hypotension, and a postural fall in blood pressure was not detected at the physical examination. Her fall was more likely to have been due to a trip, stumble or missed footing, possibly because she had not fully woken from sleep. There was probably no causal relation between the patient's "dizziness" and her fall, though the fall might have exacerbated her fear of falling.

Question E   1

The vague nature of her dizziness, its tendency to persist all day, her recent edginess and the fine tremor, all point towards anxiety. Feelings of depersonalisation and derealisation in anxiety states and depression are also sometimes described as "dizziness" by the patient. Old age is not itself a cause of dizziness.

Vertebrobasilar insufficiency is unlikely in this patient; it usually causes episodes of vertigo, which are often related to neck movements, or drop attacks.

Patients with intracranial space-occupying lesions sometimes experience dizziness, though there are usually other symptoms (such as headache) and focal neurological signs present. This patient's headaches had been present for many years and were therefore unlikely to be caused by serious intracranial pathology.

The patient's blood pressure was only mildly elevated and would not be expected to produce any symptoms. Most hypertensives do not complain of dizziness, and most patients complaining of dizziness are not hypertensive.

Question F   2

Hyperthyroidism presents in various atypical ways in the elderly. The patient's complaints, the tremor and the change in mental state could be caused by thyrotoxicosis and measurement of thyroid function should be performed.

There are no indications for any of the other investigations in this case.

Question G   3

The best way to proceed is to gather as much information as possible about the patient's well-being and behaviour from a close relative or friend. Thus it is possible to gain a better perspective of her illness.

Prescribing a tranquilliser or hypnotic might dampen her anxiety and control some of her symptoms. This is not really an adequate approach, and an attempt should be made to discover why the patient's frame of mind has recently changed. Ideally, the patient would not be referred to the psychiatrist until a relative has been interviewed, though of the remaining options, number 4 is the most reasonable. The patient's illness was mild, she has good support at home and there were no psychotic features, so admission as a psychiatric in-patient was not necessary.

Question H   3

The features of her illness suggest a mild to moderate agitated depression; anxiety is often prominent in this condition.

The depression which follows bereavement usually occurs shortly after the death of the spouse and has generally resolved within a year or so; delayed bereavement reactions occasionally occur, though not as long as 11 years later.

The patient had no history of being chronically anxious; indeed the appearance of anxiety "out of the blue" with no obvious precipitating cause should always raise the possibility of depression in the clinician's mind.

She was restless and alert, but did not have the "high" affect of a patient with hypomania.

There was no evidence of a decline in intellectual function, memory or decorum, which would have pointed towards a dementing illness.

Question I

When an elderly patient has only a mild to moderate depression, good support at home and no psychotic symptoms or suicidal ideas, it is reasonable for the geriatrician or general practitioner to prescribe an antidepressant and keep the patient under review. Tricyclic drugs are effective but have troublesome side-effects, the most important of which is postural hypotension; tetracyclic drugs appear to have fewer such side-effects. In a patient such as this, amitriptyline (a tricyclic) would be suitable because of its sedative properties, and the total daily dose can be given at night if the patient is sleeping poorly. Mianserin (a tetracyclic) could be used in the same way.

If the patient is more profoundly depressed, has marked weight loss, psychotic symptoms, suicidal ideas, severe agitation, psychomotor retardation or pseudodementia, a referral should be made to a psychiatrist, preferably one with specialist training in psychogeriatrics.

Question J   All of them.

Any one, or combination, of the options could be present. It is essential to examine the eyes thoroughly to establish the cause of failing vision, and if necessary, the opinion of an ophthalmologist should be sought.

This patient's optic fundus had the appearance of that in Figure 7.

Question K

Senile macular degeneration.

Suggested further reading

Goldstein S F (1979) Depression in the elderly. Journal of the American Geriatrics Society, 27, 38-42

Post F (1985) The central nervous system - the emotional disorders. In: Brocklehurst J C (ed.) Textbook of Geriatric Medicine and Gerontology, 3rd Edn. Churchill Livingstone, Edinburgh

CASE 10

FOUND SEMICONSCIOUS ON THE FLOOR

HISTORY

In November 1984, an elderly man who lived alone had been behaving in a strange manner for about a week, and his neighbour asked the general practitioner to visit him. Apparently, the patient had been in fairly good health until about 7-10 days before. The GP found the patient in a semiconscious state on the living room sofa. His heart rate was 50/minute and blood pressure 100/60 mmHg.

There was a history of peptic ulcer and the GP believed the patient to be a fairly heavy drinker. The patient was admitted to hospital as an urgency.

Question A

Which of these is the least likely diagnosis in this case?

1. Haemorrhage with consequent shock

2. Complete heart block

3. Hypothermia

4. Alcohol intoxication

5. Starvation

EXAMINATION

On physical examination he was unkempt and his clothes were soiled with urine and faeces, the rectal temperature was 31°C. His respiratory rate was 12, pulse 48/minute and blood pressure 90/50 mmHg. No other abnormalities were found.

Question B

Which of the following could complicate this man's hypothermia?

1. Acute renal failure

2. Pneumonia

3. Pressure sores

4. Acute pancreatitis

5. Gastrointestinal haemorrhage

Question C

Which of the following are risk factors for hypothermia?

1. Pneumonia

2. Parkinson's disease

3. Stroke

4. Dementia

5. Social isolation

Question D

Which of the following drugs could predispose a patient to hypothermia?

1. Benzodiazepines

2. Chlorpromazine

3. L-thyroxine

4. α-Methyldopa

5. Alcohol

He had no next of kin; his neighbour said the patient was well and caring for himself until a few days before admission. The patient had then started to wander half-clothed into the garden, shouted abuse at the neighbours and refused help.

Question E

Discuss the possible reasons for this abnormal behaviour.

TREATMENT

Question F

In view of this patient's condition, which of the following methods of rewarming should be used?

1. Rapid rewarming by immersion in water at 40°C.

2. Core rewarming by repetitive peritoneal lavage with warmed peritoneal dialysis fluid.

3. Allow the patient's body temperature to rise of its own accord, in a warm room, controlling the rate of rewarming by the use of blankets.

4. Warm, sweet drinks and vigorous exercise.

5. Intravenous tri-iodothyronine, a space blanket and infrared lamps.

Question G

During rewarming, at which of the following temperatures is the risk of ventricular fibrillation at its highest?

1. When the patient's body temperature is at its lowest.

2. During the "overshoot" pyrexia which sometimes occurs.

3. 30°C

4. 35°C

5. 32°C

Question H

What is thought to be the ideal rate of rewarming for elderly hypothermics?

INVESTIGATIONS

Question I

Discuss the investigations you would perform on this patient.

The patient had reached normal body temperature by the following day; he remained confused and later developed a pyrexia of 38.4°C. At this time his heart rate was 90, blood pressure 140/80 mmHg, respiratory rate 28, and no definite physical signs were found in the mouth, throat, chest or abdomen.

Question J

What is the most likely cause of the pyrexia?

After suitable treatment, he improved and his confusion resolved.

Question K

How would you organise his discharge from hospital? Which staff would you involve?

ANSWERS

Question A   1

Despite the history of peptic ulcer, it is unlikely that he has had a substantial GI haemorrhage since his heart rate is only 50.

Two and three are the most likely diagnoses, as the presentation would be in keeping and both cause hypotension and bradycardia.

Starvation is always a possible diagnosis in an elderly person living alone, though the history of him having been well just a week or so before makes this less likely.

Alcohol intoxication is worth bearing in mind in view of the background history, though intoxicated patients usually have a fairly high heart rate.

Question B   All 5

Bronchopneumonia is a relatively common sequel to hypothermia; defence against invasion of the lower respiratory tract is probably impaired when body temperature is low. In some patients, the pneumonia is probably the primary event, which may lead to confusion, wandering or falls with hypothermia as a consequence.

Acute renal failure and acute pancreatitis are by no means rare complications of hypothermia, and usually become clinically apparent after rewarming.

Pressure sores can result whenever a patient loses consciousness and remains immobile for more than about 2 hours.

Upper gastrointestinal haemorrhage is a fairly frequent post-mortem finding in hypothermics who die. It is difficult to diagnose during severe hypothermia, and is one of the causes of a persistent low blood pressure during rewarming; such patients do not usually have a haematemesis while the body temperature is low.

Question C   All 5

Any condition which predisposes a patient to falls or confusion increases the risk of hypothermia. Socially isolated patients are less likely to be found quickly if they fall, and they are less likely to summon help in the event of running out of food or if the means of heating their home fails.

Question D   1, 2, 4 and 5

Benzodiazepines can cause falls and thereby put the patient at risk from hypothermia; also, patients who are drowsy are less likely to take appropriate action to keep warm if the environmental temperature falls.

Chlorpromazine causes subcutaneous vasodilatation and reduces shivering; even modest doses can result in a fall in core temperature during cool weather.

α-Methyldopa can cause postural hypotension and thereby falls; some patients become depressed and could consequently neglect themselves and hence risk hypothermia.

Alcohol abuse is an important contributory risk factor for hypothermia by causing falls, confusion, and subcutaneous vasodilatation, as well as sometimes leading the patient to neglect proper nutrition, clothing and heating.

Question E

From the description, it is likely that he was becoming gradually more hypothermic over a number of days. Also, there was a history of probable alcohol abuse, which could have led to his unusual behaviour. However, it must be remembered that a multitude of different underlying conditions can present with confusion, altered behaviour and self-neglect in the elderly.

Question F 3

Experience has shown that most elderly hypothermics will rewarm themselves if placed in a warm environment; anecdotal evidence suggests that death is least likely to occur if this method is used.

Rapid warming by immersion in warm water has been advocated for the treatment of young people with hypothermia caused by exposure. This method has no place in the elderly, in whom it can lead to fatal cardiovascular collapse.

Rewarming by peritoneal lavage has been used in hypothermics who do not spontaneously rewarm themselves, and is particularly indicated if there is associated renal failure. This method should be performed in an intensive care unit.

Warm, sweet drinks and exercise are obviously not appropriate in a patient with a lowered level of consciousness. Intravenous triiodothyronine will only be of benefit if the patient is hypothermic due to true hypothyroidism.

Question G 5

A number of observations and studies have shown that ventricular fibrillation is most likely to occur during rewarming when the core temperature is rising through about 32°C.

Question H

Proper comparative studies have not been performed, but the collective evidence suggests that at a rate of 0.5°C per hour the risks of arrythmias and shock are at a minimum. If the blood pressure starts to fall, the rate of rewarming should be slowed down.

Question I

The patient should be disturbed as little as possible while rewarming is in progress; this probably reduces the risk of fatal arrhythmias occurring. After core (rectal) temperature has risen to over 35°C, it is advisable to measure the patient's blood glucose, urea, electrolytes and haemoglobin and to perform a chest radiograph and electrocardiogram. Thyroid function tests should be done in all hypothermics. These basic tests will provide information on the most likely consequences of hypothermia, that is, hypoglycaemia, renal impairment, electrolyte imbalance, anaemia due to gastrointestinal haemorrhage, pneumonia and cardiac arrhythmias. Other specific investigations will depend on what the patient's condition indicates; for example, if there is abdominal pain and tenderness, the serum amylase should be measured to detect pancreatitis.

Question J

Pneumonia is the likely cause of the pyrexia; it is particularly common after hypothermia, and the high respiratory rate should lead one to suspect a chest infection in this case. The absence of physical signs in the chest does not exclude the diagnosis, which will be more reliably confirmed by chest radiography. Of course, other infections can occur in this context.

Question K

It is important to ask yourself the question "Why did he become hypothermic?". There was no apparent metabolic cause, and after recovery he was not confused. A visit to his house by the medical social worker, or a home visit by the patient along with the medical social worker and, perhaps, occupational therapist, might provide an explanation, and reveal scope for preventing a recurrence. Particular note should be made of heating, food, bedclothes, and the state of windows and doors.

He should be warned of the danger of excessive alcohol intake, and it would be worthwhile arranging for the health visitor or district nurse to visit him to keep an eye on his drinking habits, and, in cold weather, to measure his body temperature. A substantial proportion of hypothermics have impaired thermoregulation, this probably precedes the first episode of overt clinical hypothermia. Such patients are at particular risk of further episodes of hypothermia and require close supervision after discharge. The cause of such thermal instability is not certain, though it is thought to be due to ageing changes in the hypothalamic thermoregulatory centre.

An offer of meals-on-wheels would ensure at least one good meal per day, and a home-help, perhaps weekly, could make sure he had food in the house, and that his heating was reasonable.

Suggested further reading

British Medical Journal: Leading Article (1978) Treating accidental hypothermia. British Medical Journal, **2**, 1381-84

Maclean D, Eanslie-Smith D (1977) Accidental Hypothermia. Blackwell Scientific Publications, Oxford, London

CASE 11

CONTINUING CARE

HISTORY

Mr T R, a 76-year-old widower, had his third stroke, a left hemiparesis, in December 1984. He had had two right hemipareses in 1983, and had made a sufficiently good recovery to enable him to live alone with support from an aged, partially-sighted sister, who lived nearby, a home-help and a bath nurse. He had no other living relatives.

He was unable to stand and had become incontinent of urine. His general practitioner arranged for him to be admitted to hospital urgently.

Question A

After initial assessment in the admission room, which of the following should he do?

1. Go directly to the rehabilitation ward.

2. Go directly to a continuing care ward.

3. Be admitted to an acute assessment ward.

PHYSICAL CONDITION 3 WEEKS AFTER ADMISSION TO THE ASSESSMENT WARD

He had not improved neurologically or functionally since admission. He was dysarthric, unable to feed himself, unable to stand without the support of two people and incontinent of urine. There was power reduction to 2/5 in both arms, and 4/5 in the right leg, and 3/5 in the left leg. He was hypertonic in all four limbs. He had very poor truncal balance, left-sided sensory neglect and a left homonymous hemianopia. His short-term memory was poor.

Question B

These are your main options; which would you choose in this case?

1. Transfer him to your stroke rehabilitation ward for intensive physiotherapy.

2. Transfer him to a slow-stream rehabilitation bed with a view to discharge after several months.

3. Transfer him to a continuing care (long-stay) ward.

4.   Discharge him with a wheelchair and maximal social services support at home.

5.   Keep him in the assessment ward for at least 3 more weeks before making a decision.

The patient was transferred to a long-stay ward containing 16 beds in four bays. The ward contained a mixture of demented and sensible, physically disabled patients.

He was placed in a bay with three other men, all of whom were able to hold a rational conversation with him. After 2 weeks he started to refuse his food and would not talk to his fellow patients. There was nothing new to find on physical examination.

Question C

The most likely reason for this change is:

1.   A further stroke

2.   An endogenous depression

3.   A reactive depression similar to bereavement

4.   Multi-infarct dementia

5.   A paranoid psychosis

The patient's urinary incontinence was associated with severe urgency of micturition; he had no dribbling incontinence between. His urine was sterile and his prostate gland normal on rectal examination.

Question D

What would be your initial approach to the management of the patient's urinary incontinence?

PROGRESS

Two months after admission the patient's mood had improved considerably. His incontinence was under control and he was taking no medication. The physiotherapist had seen him regularly to perform passive exercises to reduce his hypertonia and avoid limb contractures. It was not difficult for two people to transfer him from bed to chair. His family were very keen to take him home for a couple of days over Christmas; this was arranged. Unfortunately, when he returned to the ward he had developed an area of pressure necrosis over the sacrum, and he had frequent soiling of his clothes with semi-liquid faeces.

Question E

The skin over the pressure ulcer was blackened (8 cm diameter) and beginning to separate. Answer the following:

1. For how long can tissue be safely compressed before there is risk of ischaemic necrosis?

2. What factors determine the amount of pressure required to cause necrosis?

3. How would you avoid extending the area of necrosis?

4. How might you remove the eschar and underlying necrotic tissue?

5. What methods promote healing and epithelialisation of the pressure sore?

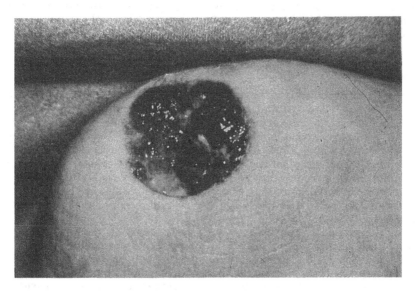

Figure 8 Pressure sore

Question F

The pressure sore in Figure 8 is from another patient. What phase of healing is it in? How could you speed up complete healing?

Question G

What is the likely cause of his faecal incontinence? How would you confirm your diagnosis and how would you treat it?

Within 10 weeks the pressure sore had healed completely. The patient had come to feel more at home on the ward and expressed a wish to take part in a number of activities organised for the long-stay patients. His incontinence of urine was controlled sufficiently well to enable him to keep his personal clothes in good condition. He died of pneumonia 8 months later.

ANSWERS

Question A 3

Acutely ill elderly patients should almost always be placed in an assessment ward in the first instance, even if it seems likely that they will eventually require rehabilitation or continuing care. Thus, the medical aspects of their acute illness can be investigated and treated more quickly and effectively. Some departments have separate acute, rehabilitation and long-stay wards, and others have various types of mixed wards; however, the same general principle of admitting such patients to an assessment bed still applies. This policy also enables a proper judgement as to whether the patient would benefit from a trial of rehabilitation or not.

Question B 3

Option 3 is probably the best on balance, though there is some room for debate. The patient is unlikely to benefit from intensive rehabilitation, and is very unlikely to be independent again, in view of his severe bilateral power loss, poor balance, sensory inattention on the left, visual field defect and lack of reliable home support. The absence of any improvement during the 3 weeks of assessment also indicates a poor outcome. A case could be made for a trial of slow stream rehabilitation, though it would probably be better to transfer the patient directly to a continuing care ward and settle him down there.

He would not be able to survive at home as he was unable to move from a wheelchair, unable to operate the wheelchair because of the weakness of his arms, and unable to feed or toilet himself. His sister was too frail to provide the necessary nursing care.

Little would be gained from a further period of assessment, and the patient would be occupying a bed required for an acutely ill patient.

Question C 3

Patients who have recently suffered from a disabling stroke frequently become depressed, particularly when they see little or no improvement in their condition. The impact of such a depressing event can often be reduced by sympathetic but optimistic handling by nurses and other staff, or by recreational activities, clubs, outings and the like. Antidepressant drugs are sometimes required. Most patients' mood will improve within a few weeks.

A further stroke would usually be accompanied by fresh physical signs, and be of sudden onset.

Endogenous depression could occur in this context, though there would usually be a history of depressive or manic depressive illness.

Patients with multi-infarct dementia would not usually exhibit a gradual withdrawal over a 2-week period; a step-wise reduction in intellectual power, disinhibition and patchy bilateral hypertonia are the usual features.

A paranoid psychosis could present with withdrawal in the early stages, though this patient had no first rank psychotic symptoms.

Question D

The nature of the patient's urinary incontinence is suggestive of an uninhibited neurogenic bladder probably, in this case, due to his severe cerebrovascular disease. A reasonable way to deal with this would be to toilet him regularly, say 2-hourly, so that his bladder is emptied before it reaches the volume which causes urgency. Regular toiletting at night often helps to prevent or reduce nocturnal incontinence. Avoiding drinks in the evening also helps. Drugs can be used to reduce frequency in these circumstances; in this patient's case it might be possible to utilise the anticholinergic side-effects of a tricyclic antidepressant drug for this purpose, if it is thought necessary to treat his depression with drugs.

At this stage, a urinary catheter should be avoided.

Question E

1. It is known from animal experiments and clinic experience that sustained pressure which results in capillary occlusion for less than 2 hours does not result in tissue necrosis, whereas sustained pressure for 7 hours or more invariably leads to some tissue damage. For clinical purposes, an upper limit of 2 hours should be assumed; hence the need for frequent turning of immobile patients.

2. To cause necrosis, pressure within the tissue must be sustained at a level above mean capillary perfusion pressure (about 25 mmHg). Small blood vessels can also be occluded by folding or shearing of the skin, such as tends to occur over the buttocks and sacrum when a patient is sliding down from the semi-recumbent position in bed.

    If tissue perfusion is poor, or the blood pressure low, then capillary flow will cease at even lower pressures.

    The amount of pressure at points over an area depends on the patient's weight and the size of the surface area over which it is distributed. Hence, for an average sized man, the pressures over the occiput, sacrum and heel whilst lying on a foam mattress are about 50, 60 and 50 mmHg respectively, all of which exceed mean capillary perfusion pressure.

3. Once a pressure sore has occurred it is essential to prevent extension of it by avoiding further sustained pressure in the area, or other areas. Other risk factors such as anaemia, malnutrition, hypotension, septicaemia, etc. should also be dealt with as quickly as possible. In other words, all the measures to **prevent** pressure sores should be started.

4. Whilst some healing will occur below a clean eschar, the ulcer will not epithelialise properly until it is removed. Some eschars detach spontaneously; others require surgical removal. A useful method which can be performed in the ward is to infiltrate the space immediately below the eschar with a solution containing the proteolytic enzymes streptokinase and streptodornase; these lyse the protein bonds between the eschar and the underlying tissue and facilitate its removal. Minor surgical debridement of residual eschar may be necessary in some cases.

   Eusol and similar agents help in the removal of necrotic debris but should not be applied to clean granulation tissue, which can be damaged by them with a consequent prolongation of ulcer healing time.

5. Methods of proven benefit are few and relatively straightforward. These include prevention of further pressure necrosis, removal of necrotic tissue, keeping the ulcer as clean as possible (though it can never be sterile), treatment to improve the patient's nutritional status and correction of anaemia. Patience is required.

Antibiotics are not of established benefit when applied locally, though they will be needed if healthy tissue adjacent to the ulcer becomes infected or if the patient becomes septicaemic.

Dressings which conform to the ulcer shape are useful (e.g. Debrisan) but tight packing should be avoided as this can actually cause further pressure necrosis. Skin grafting speeds up epithelialisation.

A vast array of other remedies have been advocated, such as ultraviolet light, local insulin, chlorophyll, high dose vitamin C, anabolic steroids, ozone, oxygen and so on. None of these is supported by reliable evidence of therapeutic benefit. Honey dressings probably do help by providing a very high osmotic pressure which dehydrates bacteria, prevents their multiplication and thereby reduces the bacterial load within the ulcer.

Question F

This is a pressure sore which has been properly cared for so that a large amount of viable granulation tissue has grown in from its edges and base. Very little residual necrotic tissue is present. The blood supply is likely to be good. This ulcer, though at an advanced stage of healing, would require several weeks to be covered by epithelium growing in from the edges. A split-skin graft would markedly reduce the time for epithelialisation in this case.

Question G

This type of faecal incontinence is usually caused by severe constipation with faecal impaction and consequent overflow of frequent small volumes of liquid faeces. Immobile patients are particularly prone to this. Digital examination of the rectum will confirm the diagnosis. Treatment is by repeated enemata until the rectum is empty; this method is successful in the majority of cases. It is important to prevent recurrence by giving a laxative of the bulk-forming or stool-softening type. Regular enemata are sometimes needed.

Suggested further reading

Agate J N (1985) Aging and the skin - pressure sores. In: Brocklehurst J C (ed.) Textbook of Geriatric Medicine and Gerontology, 3rd Edn. Churchill Livingstone, Edinburgh

Andrews J (1981) Prevention and care of pressure sores. In: Andrews J and Von Hahn (eds.) Geriatrics for Everyday Practice. Karger, Basle

Bigot A, Mannicks J M A (1985) The psychology of long-term and terminal illness in old age. In: Brocklehurst J C (ed.) Textbook of Geriatric Medicine and Gerontology, 3rd Edn. Churchill Livingstone, Edinburgh

CASE 12

A DANGER TO HIMSELF AND OTHERS

HISTORY

You are telephoned by the neighbour of a patient on a Saturday evening. Apparently, the patient has been shouting at passers-by from his bedroom window, using obscene language, and has been throwing faeces at children who tease him. He has led a reclusive life for many years, though until recently had not made a nuisance of himself. A week before, the fire brigade had to come and extinguish a fire he started in the shed at the side of his house. His records showed that he has not consulted a doctor for many years. He has no known relatives.

When you arrive, the patient refuses to allow you in or to reason with you in any way. You learn from the neighbour that the Area Social Worker has also been unable to gain entry.

The patient spits at you through the letter box and announces that he wants to be left alone to "do away with himself".

Question A

You feel a compulsory admission is justified. Why?

Which section of the Public Assistance Act (1947) enables you to proceed, and how would you arrange this?

The patient was admitted to an acute psychogeriatric bed after consultation with the psychogeriatrician. A diagnosis of severe agitated depression with paranoid ideas was made. Routine haematological and biochemical tests were normal.

Question B

True or false?

1. Elderly patients with agitated depression rarely kill themselves.

2. When paranoid ideas are well formed, the diagnosis of depression is in doubt.

3. Depression and dementia rarely co-exist.

4. Electroconvulsive therapy is often effective in severe depression in old age.

5. Depression is not strongly related to intelligence.

Question C

True or false?

Electroconvulsive therapy is usually contraindicated:

1. In patients with stable angina of effort
2. 4 weeks after a stroke
3. In all patients with Alzheimer's disease
4. When a patient is taking digoxin
5. If the diastolic blood pressure is 120 mmHg or more

Question D

Discuss how you would tackle the following problems in this patient.

1. Daytime sedation while he is still very agitated.
2. Night-time sedation.
3. Sedation at a time when the patient had an otherwise uncontrollable outburst of anger and agitation, struck out at the nursing staff and threatened to kill himself.

The patient made a steady recovery from his depression and returned to his pre-morbid rational, but rather reclusive, frame of mind.

Question E

How would you plan his discharge and follow-up?

ANSWERS

Question A

The man is clearly very disturbed, he has acted violently towards others and is possibly a danger to those living nearby. He has probably either accidently or purposely started a fire, and he has threatened suicide; he is therefore likely to be a danger to himself. He evidently will not consider an informal admission, so a compulsory admission is reasonable in this case.

A patient such as this can be admitted by use of Section 47 of the Public Assistance Act (1947). The patient's general practitioner or a hospital doctor should first contact the District Community Physician. Evidence is then presented by the local Health Authority to a Magistrate, who can give an "order" for the patient to be taken to a hospital or other public institution for assessment. The order lasts for 48 hours and can be renewed. Compulsory admission should be avoided whenever possible.

Other types of compulsory admission and treatment are occasionally required. The advice of a psychiatrist should be sought as early as possible.

Question B   4 and 5 are true.

The elderly tolerate electroconvulsive therapy fairly well, and the method is often very successful in severe depression.

People of all levels of intelligence can become depressed, though the patient's intellectual and cultural background may colour the illness in various ways.

The elderly with agitated depression are particularly prone to suicide. Well formed paranoid ideas are not rare in endogenous depression, and probably enhance the suicide risk.

Depression and dementia are both common and, not infrequently, are both present in one patient. This can create diagnostic difficulties and it is good policy to seek the opinion of a psychogeriatrician in such cases.

Question C   2 and 5 are true.

Most psychiatrists avoid using ECT within 6 months of a stroke as there is thought to be a risk of haemorrhage into the area of brain infarction during the transient, but considerable, rise in blood pressure which occurs during the induced convulsion.

The main risks of ECT when the patient is hypertensive are those associated with the anaesthesia; uncontrolled hypertensives are more prone to cerebral and myocardial infarction during anaesthesia. The usual practice is to bring the blood pressure down to a reasonable level (say a diastolic of less than 110 mmHg) before starting ECT.

Stable angina is not a contraindication; the patients are well oxygenated during ECT. Patients with severe unstable angina may be at risk of myocardial infarction or fatal arrhythmias under these circumstances. Recent myocardial infarction is a contraindication as fatal arrhythmias can occur.

Patients with mild to moderate Alzheimer's dementia who are depressed can be given ECT if necessary, though the transient confusion which often follows ECT in the elderly can be troublesome in such patients. Those with more advanced dementia do not tolerate ECT well.

Digoxin is not a contraindication; indeed, patients with uncontrolled atrial fibrillation should be digitalised before having ECT. However, those with digoxin toxicity might develop serious arrhythmias during ECT.

Question D

1.   Once the diagnosis of depression is made, an antidepressant drug can be given, and if agitation is a troublesome feature, a drug with sedative properties, such as amitriptyline or dothiepin should be used. When anxiety colours the agitation a benzodiazepine often helps; the aim is to take the "edge" off the anxiety without producing too much drowsiness. Phenothiazines, such as chlorpromazine or thioridazine, can be used in a similar way.

2. Sedation at night in these circumstances can often be achieved by giving the largest dose of a b.d. or t.d.s. regimen of amitriptyline at night, or the whole dose of mianserin at night. If insomnia is a feature, the choice of sedation will depend on the pattern of the sleeplessness; benzodiazepines are particularly effective when anxiety is prominent at night, though large doses of long-acting ones, such as nitrazepam, can result in excessive residual sedation next morning and the short-acting preparations, for example, temazepam, sometimes result in abrupt awakening of the patient in the early hours of the morning as plasma levels are falling. Chloral hydrate and triclofos are useful alternatives, and are probably the drugs of choice when anxiety is not prominent.

3. When the patient has otherwise uncontrollable outbursts of agitation and anger, drugs may be needed to rapidly sedate him. He is unlikely to agree to take an oral preparation. Intravenous diazepam is effective, though difficult to administer in these circumstances. Deep intramuscular injections of chlorpromazine or haloperidol are tried and tested in this context. Care should be taken to given a substantial enough dose to achieve adequate sedation; if too little is given the patient may become even less controllable, and this then leads to a second uncomfortable injection. Postural hypotension can occur. Paraldehyde is effective, though painful and irritant when injected, hence it is rarely used except when patients are very prone to cardiovascular side-effects when given phenothiazines.

Question E

Firstly, a decision has to be made as to whether the patient can realistically manage to live alone; if there is doubt about this the occupational therapists should make an "activities of daily living" (ADL) assessment. The medical social worker should visit the house well beforehand to see what condition it is in and, if necessary, arrange for the social services to have it cleaned up and made habitable. Support services, if needed, should be set up so that they start as soon as the patient is discharged.

The general practitioner should be informed of the discharge a few days in advance. The community psychiatric nurse (if available) or district nurse, should call frequently at first to look for signs of relapse and to supervise his drug regimen. Psychiatric follow-up in outpatients will be necessary; psychogeriatricians often prefer to do follow-up visits in the patient's home.

Suggested further reading

Bluglass R (1983) A Guide to the Mental Health Act. Churchill Livingstone, Edinburgh, Edinburgh

Frazer R M (1981) ECT and the elderly. In: Palmer R L (ed) Electroconvulsive Therapy, an Appraisal. Oxford University Press

Wells C E (1980) The differential diagnosis of psychiatric disorders in the elderly. In: Cole J O and Bennett J E (eds.) Psychopathology in the Aged. Raven Bros, New York

Williamson J (1978) Depression in the elderly. Age and Ageing, 7 (Suppl), 35-44

CASE 13

WEAK PAINFUL LEGS

HISTORY AND EXAMINATION

A 71-year-old woman was referred to hospital by her general practitioner because she was unable to rise from her wheelchair. Several years previously she had been investigated for aches and pains; radiographs of her joints showed only cervical spondylosis and her rheumatoid factor was negative. She had been treated with a variety of analgesics. Eighteen months ago she had been prescribed a wheelchair and she had been chairfast for a year. She had not been out of the house for many years. Admission was precipitated by the fact that her husband could no longer lift her. Her drugs were: Navidrex-K (cyclopenthiazide + Slow-K), 2 tablets daily, benorylate, 4 g three times daily, nitrazepam, 5 mg nightly and an aperient.

On admission she was complaining of pain in her legs which was localised around the knees. There were hard lumps on the front of both shins and the dorsal aspects of the forearms and marked bowing of the tibias. She was unable to raise her legs from the bed, and the tendon jerks were not elicitable (though they were normal in the arms). There was no sensory disturbance apart from blunted vibration sense at the ankles. The plantar responses were flexor, and dorsiflexion and plantar-flexion were of normal power. Movements of the fingers, wrists, shoulders and hips were full and pain-free. She was a vegan and was thin, weighing only 42 kg. Initial investigations showed: Hb 8.2 g/dl, MCV 76 fl, ESR 56 mm/hour.

Question A

Which of the following are true of elderly patients with polyarthritis?

1. Heberden's nodes are a reliable indicator in distinguishing rheumatoid arthritis from osteoarthritis.

2. Subcutaneous nodules are highly suggestive of active rheumatoid disease.

3. A diagnosis of rheumatoid arthritis can usually be made by the typical changes in the hands.

4. Rheumatoid arthritis is uncommon in the elderly, and is nearly always a low-grade process extending over many years.

5. Positive tests for rheumatoid factor indicate active disease.

75

Further investigations showed:

Serum B_{12} 325 ng/l

RBC folate 125 μg/l

TIBC 90 μmol/l
   (saturation = 4.4%)

Urea 9.8 mmol/l

Bicarbonate 19 mmol/l

Phosphate 0.7 mmol/l

Albumin 42 g/l

Alkaline phosphatase 378 iu/l

Serum folate 1.7 μg/l

Serum iron 4 μmol/l

2 of 3 faecal occult blood tests
   positive

Creatinine 0.08 mmol/l

Calcium 2.34 mmol/l

Glucose 6.0 mmol/l

Globulin 45 g/l

Aspartate transaminase 11 iu/l

Radiographs of her hips and knees showed mild changes of osteo-arthrosis. All her drugs were stopped. One week later her urea was 10.5 mmol/l and it remained at this level, but the other biochemical tests did not change.

Question B

Discuss

1. Why could she not walk?

2. Give one factor which may have caused the low serum bicar-bonate.

3. Does she have renal impairment (urea 10.5 mmol/l; creatinine 0.08 mmol/l)?

4. What is the single most likely cause of a raised alkaline phos-phatase in an elderly patient?

5. Are there any other significant abnormalities in the biochemi-cal tests?

FURTHER MANAGEMENT

Radiographs of the pelvis and femora showed gross changes of osteomalacia (see Figure 9) and no vitamin D could be detected in her serum. She was treated with 1-α-cholecalciferol (alphacalcidol), 2 μg intramuscularly daily, and oral calcium, 1 g per day, and made a slow but steady improvement. Although her corrected free serum calcium returned to normal in 3 months, her pseudo-fractures remained radiologically non-united for many months and the alkaline phosphatase did not fall for over a year. Her anaemia was shown to be due to iron deficiency and was reversed by oral supplements; the serum folate was also slightly reduced.

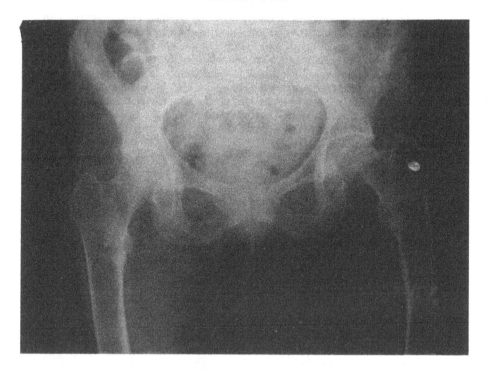

Figure 9 Osteomalacia

Question C

Discuss

1.   Was the prescription of 1-α-hydroxycholecalciferol correct in this case?

2.   What other therapy could have been given?

3.   Give two likely important factors in the aetiology of her osteomalacia.

4.   "Lack of diarrhoea makes malabsorption unlikely": true or false?

5.   Is a bone biopsy the only definitive way of establishing a diagnosis of osteomalacia in the elderly?

ANSWERS

Question A   2 and 3

Heberden's nodes are common in the elderly, and thus are of little help in deciding either the severity of generalised osteoarthritis or in excluding rheumatoid arthritis. Subcutaneous nodules have the same significance as in the young (i.e. highly suggestive of active rheumatoid arthritis). While it is true that rheumatoid arthritis can often be diagnosed by inspection of the hands (see Figure 10), hands may not be so helpful: (a) early in the course of the disease; and (b) when the rheumatoid process is affecting predominantly extra-articular tissues. Rheumatoid arthritis is common in the elderly, and not infrequently cripples within a few years. Florid disease may start in the 70s or 80s, but be missed because of the apparent lack of constitutional symptoms and signs. Up to 25% of the elderly may have positive tests for rheumatoid factor.

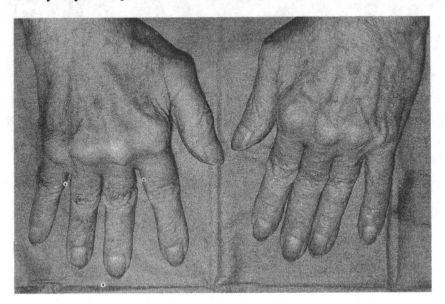

Figure 10 An example of non-florid seropositive rheumatoid arthritis which began at the age of 74

Question B

1. She could not walk because of muscular weakness. The absence of other neurological signs, and the relative strength of the calf and tibial muscles suggest a proximal myopathy.

2. She is on a high dose of an aspirin-like drug (the equivalent of 7.2 g/day aspirin). She is small and has poor renal function, and thus may have chronic salicylate toxicity. Renal tubular acidosis may occasionally be found.

3. She is likely to have renal impairment. The serum creatinine is "normal" but she is very small, and will have a low muscle mass, which will result in a low creatinine. It is well recognised that, for this reason, creatinine may be normal in the elderly, even when the glomerular filtration rate is less than 50 ml min^{-1} 1.72 m^{-2}; a urea of 10 mmol/l is consistent with this.

4. Paget's disease of the bone is probably the commonest cause of a raised alkaline phosphatase in the elderly, particularly if it is the sole biochemical abnormality.

5. Yes: her calculated free serum calcium is low (1.25 nmol/l, reference range 1.33-1.55 in elderly female patients). Both the albumin and globulin were high in this patient which obscures the low free calcium. Abnormalities of the albumin concentration are common in elderly patients, and should be borne in mind when assessing total calcium values.

Question C

1. Alphacalcidol offers no advantage over calciferol in patients with reasonable renal function; it is more expensive than cholecalciferol, and carries a higher risk of hypercalcaemia, particularly if extra oral calcium is given.

2. A single injection of 7.5 mg of cholecalciferol (300 000 units) may be used as a complete replacement dose, and has been shown to be effective and safe in the elderly. Exposure to artificial ultraviolet light has also been shown to be effective, but is more time consuming.

3. Risk factors for this patient were an inadequate diet (she was a vegan, and took neither meat nor fortified margarines), and lack of direct exposure to summer sunlight (she always sunbathed behind glass).

4. False: diarrhoea may be absent even in severe malabsorption especially if the serum calcium is low. The elderly may have mild forms of malabsorption due to bacterial overgrowth in the small bowel without alteration in bowel habit.

5. When florid radiological changes are present they may be diagnostic of osteomalacia, otherwise bone biopsy is the only definitive method. Serum vitamin D assays are less helpful in the old than in the young because there is a considerable overlap between "normals" and those with biopsy-proven osteomalacia. Serum phosphate is often paradoxically high because of the decline in renal function, and the alkaline phosphatase is commonly raised for other reasons. Changes in serum calcium may be quite mild, which is why it is helpful to calculate the free calcium.

Suggested further reading

Exton-Smith A N (1985) The musculoskeletal system - bone aging and metabolic bone disease. In: Brocklehurst J C (ed.) Textbook of Geriatric Medicine and Gerontology, 3rd Edn. Churchill Livingstone, Edinburgh

Hodkinson M (1984) Clinical Biochemistry of the Elderly. Churchill Livingstone, Edinburgh

CASE 14

PYREXIA AND A SWOLLEN LEG

HISTORY

A 76-year-old man was admitted to hospital with swelling of the whole of the left leg which had come on over a 1 week period. For 4 days he had been expectorating pink frothy sputum, and for the previous 2 nights had been sweaty. He thought that he had lost weight recently. He was said to have had a femoral vein thrombosis on the right side 10 years ago, and an episode of bronchopneumonia 6 months before admission. He had also had a proven myocardial infarction in the past.

EXAMINATION

On examination he was afebrile but dyspnoeic. There was ankle and sacral oedema, the jugular venous pressure was elevated, the apex beat was in the 5th intercostal space, in the mid-clavicular line, and there was an ejection systolic murmur. A few coarse crepitations were present in the chest. The whole of the left leg was swollen by pitting oedema. There were no masses palpable in the groins, abdomen or pelvis (on rectal examination). Bilateral chronic ear drum perforations were noted but there was no aural discharge.

Question A

Which of the following statements are true?

1. He should be given a diuretic for his congestive cardiac failure.

2. Anticoagulants are hazardous and should not be used in the elderly.

3. Blood gases are useful in the diagnosis of pulmonary embolism in older patients.

4. Venography is only rarely indicated to prove a DVT in the old.

5. This patient is at a high risk of a major pulmonary embolus.

INVESTIGATIONS

The chest radiograph showed a small area of consolidation in the periphery of the right mid zone. The heart size was within normal limits. The ECG showed ST depression over the left ventricle. Hb 10.8 g/dl, WBC 18.7 x 10^9/l, urea 10.2 mmol/l, bilirubin 16 µmol/l, albumin 25 g/l, globulin 41 g/l.

Question B

Which of the following tests indicate diagnoses other than, or additional to, pulmonary embolism?

1. ECG (ST depression over the left ventricle).

2. Haemoglobin (10.8 g/dl).

3. Total white cell count (18.7 x 10^9/l).

4. Urea (10.2 mmol/l).

5. Serum albumin (25 g/l).

PROGRESS

A clinical diagnosis of femoral vein thrombosis and pulmonary embolism was made and the patient was anticoagulated with intravenous heparin and an oral coumarin preparation. Two weeks after this, while under good anticoagulant control, his haemoglobin fell to 8.8 g/dl and three stool occult blood tests were positive. Upper GI endoscopy was normal, and after stopping the anti-coagulants, faecal blood loss ceased.

On the fourth day in hospital he had a single temperature reading of 38°C. A blood culture taken at this time grew <u>Staph. aureus</u> as did seven further cultures when he was afebrile. A midstream specimen of urine contained 10 WBC and 20 RBC per mm^3, and echocardiography showed a poorly functioning left ventricle, and multiple echoes from the aortic root suggestive of vegetations. The serum C3 complement component was low.

Question C

Which of the following are true of infective endocarditis in the elderly?

1. <u>Staph. aureus</u> is an uncommon cause.

2. Backache may be a feature.

3. The elderly account for about a quarter of all cases, and for the majority of the mortality from this condition.

4. Females are more commonly affected than males.

5. The mitral valve is more commonly affected than the aortic.

The patient was treated with intravenous benzyl-penicillin, initially 12 g/day, and made a slow but uneventful recovery, the haemoglobin and serum albumin returning to normal over 3 months. He did, however, require maintenance therapy with diuretics for heart failure.

Question D

Which of the following statements are true about the management of endocarditis in the elderly?

1. Oral penicillin is rarely adequate for treatment of endocarditis.

2. If a rash occurs during penicillin therapy it is mandatory to change to another antibiotic.

3. The sudden onset of severe cardiac failure should first lead you to suspect a coincident myocardial infarction.

4. Purulent sputum, or a urinary tract infection, should be treated with an appropriate antibiotic.

5. Unlike younger patients, after completing therapy, future prophylaxis is rarely necessary.

ANSWERS

Question A   5 is correct.

The clinical examination suggests right ventricular failure, not congestive cardiac failure. When right heart failure is due to pulmonary embolism, diuretics should be used with caution as the cardiac output may fall precipitately. Anticoagulants are hazardous, but are commonly indicated in elderly patients, and carefully managed, present no major problems in cooperative patients. A normal arterial pO_2 may exclude a significant pulmonary embolus, but the elderly often have a slightly low pO_2 which leads to diagnostic confusion. Venography is still regarded by many as the definitive test in establishing the diagnosis of DVT and assessing its extent; it can be performed as readily in the elderly as in the young. 50% of patients with a femoral vein DVT may develop pulmonary embolism (assessed by pulmonary angiography).

Question B   2, 3, 4 and 5 are correct.

ECG changes after pulmonary embolism are often non- specific, particularly in the elderly who commonly have co-existing ischaemic heart disease. Thus, acute left ventricular ischaemia may be precipitated by a pulmonary embolus if it is big enough to cause a reduction in cardiac output. The other tests are not directly related to a pulmonary embolus and suggest that there is a chronic underlying disorder. The haemoglobin may fall if there is massive pulmonary haemorrhage (not observed in this case). The white cell count may be elevated by a pulmonary infarction itself (up to 15×10^9/l) or if a pulmonary infarct becomes secondarily infected. The elevated blood urea might have been caused by a number of conditions, as might the low serum albumin. The latter, however, strongly suggests that there has been a relatively long-standing illness.

Question C 2 and 3 are correct.

Staph. aureus has been shown quite frequently to cause subacute endocarditis in the elderly; in the young, this organism is more commonly associated with acute endocarditis. The proportion of infections due to Strep. viridans is reduced because of increased incidence of Strep. faecalis. Backache is an unexplained but frequent feature of this disorder. Over the last 30 years there has been a striking rise in the age incidence of endocarditis, the peak having moved from 20-30 years to 60-70 years old. The vast majority of deaths from this condition occur among the elderly. Despite the higher numbers of females surviving to old age, endocarditis in the elderly is commoner among males. The aortic valve is the most common site for infection in old people.

Question D 4 is correct.

Phenoxymethyl-penicillin is rapidly excreted by tubular secretion in the kidneys. This mechanism tends to be somewhat reduced in the elderly, thus higher blood levels are achieved for the same dose. Tubular secretion can be competitively blocked by probencid. In this subject, a combination of phenoxymethyl-penicillin and probencid produced trough serum levels which were inhibitory to the cultured Staph. aureus at a more than 256 dilution. Careful monitoring of therapy in this way is mandatory in all patients. Cutaneous allergy to penicillin, which occurred in this case, was controlled with an antihistamine and a corticosteroid. Myocardial infarction may occur, for example as a result of a fragmented vegetation lodging in a coronary artery, but it is vital to consider valve rupture. This may produce profound cardiac failure with little change in the murmur, especially when the aortic valve is affected. Surgery may be life-saving and should be considered. The elderly not uncommonly develop intercurrent infections, for example in the chest and urinary tract, while in hospital. Recurrence of fever during antimicrobial therapy may be due to a second infection; this should be treated accordingly. Any patient recovering from endocarditis should be regarded as liable to further attacks. Antibiotic prophylaxis should therefore be considered at the time of dental work, gastrointestinal endoscopy, urinary catheterisation and other invasive procedures. It is not clear whether elderly subjects with heart murmurs, but who have not had endocarditis, should be offered prophylaxis in similar circumstances. Some authorities recommend antibiotic prophylaxis for all such procedures in old people with aortic ejection murmurs.

Suggested further reading

Dalton M J (1984) Septicaemia and infective endocarditis. In: Fox R A (ed.) Immunology and Infection in the Elderly. Churchill Livingstone, Edinburgh

Nielson H K et al (1981) 178 fatal cases of pulmonary embolism in a medical department. Acta Medica Scandinavica, **209**, 351-35

CASE 15

ANAEMIA — 1

PRESENTATION

An 84-year-old woman was referred to outpatients in 1985 with the following letter:

"Her symptoms and examination are geriatrically vague, and she has requested a second opinion.

Twelve days ago she walked as far as the surgery but 'collapsed' outside. I ran her home by car.

Her symptoms are:

Loss of confidence for going out

Indigestion

Flatulence

Sore mouth

Biliousness

Backache

Dry skin

Itching"

The hospital records revealed the following:

1974 Investigated for heartburn and indigestion

1979 Bright red rectal bleeding; haemorrhoids diagnosed

1980 Heartburn and indigestion, nothing seen on gastroscopy

1981 Multiple consultations for indigestion

Question A

1.   Give five causes of such a "collapse" on exertion, not necessarily involving loss of consciousness.

2.   Give two causes of itching when there is no obvious rash.

EXAMINATION AND INITIAL INVESTIGATIONS

She was fully orientated, nervous, with a smooth tongue (mouth otherwise normal) (Figure 11), and slightly pale conjunctivae.

Haemoglobin 6.0 g/dl, MCV 55 fl, MCH 16 pg, MCHC 28.6 g/dl.

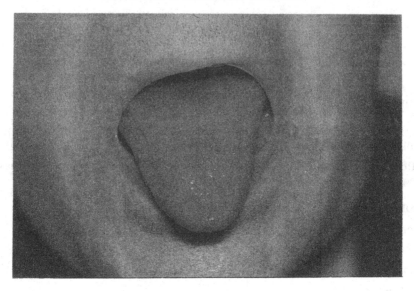

Figure 11 The patient's tongue

Question B

Discuss:

1. Why might she have been only "slightly pale" with a haemoglobin of 6 g/dl?

2. The haemoglobin falls with age and readings between 10 and 12 g/dl are not uncommon - do you agree?

3. She clearly has an iron deficiency anaemia and further investigations are probably unnecessary. Do you agree?

4. Should the serum B_{12} and folate be measured?

5. At what rate would you expect the haemoglobin to rise after starting oral iron supplements? Would this be quicker after parenteral iron?

MANAGEMENT AND PROGRESS

The serum iron was 3 µmol/l and the TIBC 93 µmol/l (3.2% saturation), confirming iron deficiency. The following tests were all normal or negative: serum B_{12}, folate and albumin, stool occult blood (x 3), sigmoidoscopy and barium enema. Upper GI endoscopy showed mild oesophagitis but no evidence of ulceration or bleeding.

She was transfused with two units of packed cells (post transfusion Hb 9.5 g/dl), given ferrous sulphate three times daily and discharged after 15 days in hospital. The Hb subsequently returned to normal, and the itching resolved.

Question C

Discuss:

1. In view of the above results, what extra information would you have liked?

2. In a similar patient, who has been investigated with negative results, what conditions might be the cause of occult bleeding?

3. For what reasons would you transfuse an elderly anaemic patient?

4. What risks of intravenous iron are of special relevance to the elderly?

ANSWERS

Question A

1. A "collapse" is a typically vague symptom among the old. In the absence of loss of consciousness, any cause which exhausts the patient's cardiorespiratory reserve may result in her simply coming to a standstill in the street. The physical signs at rest may not be very striking. Examples include asthma, emphysema, ischaemic heart disease, aortic valve disease (when syncope can also occur) and, of course, anaemia.

2. Perhaps the commonest cause of itching is a dry skin, but though fairly uncommon as a cause of itching, iron deficiency should not be forgotten.

Question B

1. Blepharitis may obscure pallor from anaemia. Conversely, the conjunctivae may be unusually pale in the presence of heart failure, even when the patient is not anaemic.

2. The normal Hb for the healthy elderly is: men 14.3 g/dl (12.3-16.2 g/dl); women 13.3 g/dl (11.5-15.1 g/dl). There may be a small age-related decline, but the mean Hb for a man aged 90 is 13.6 g/dl. A Hb below 12 g/dl in a man, and 11.5 g/dl in a woman, is clearly abnormal and requires an explanation.

3. Only iron deficiency is likely to produce the severe hypochromic/microcytic anaemia seen here. Thalassaemia would have to be considered in a younger subject but is unlikely with such a low MCHC (an acquired thalassaemia-like syndrome is a rarity and probably neoplastic). Similarly, sideroblastic anaemia, and anaemia of chronic disorders, would not produce such profound hypochromia and microcytosis. Iron deficiency may be multifactorial in the elderly; relatively low iron stores to start with, borderline diet, reduced absorption; increased

loss by desquamation and microscopic occult bleeding, and macroscopic bleeding. How far to pursue a diagnosis may be problematic in individual cases, but it seems to us that the following is an irreducible minimum:

(a) Confirm the diagnosis (serum Fe and TIBC or serum ferritin), and perform a bone marrow examination if the TIBC saturation is not low.

(b) Take a full history and physical examination including recto-sigmoidoscopy.

(c) Consider whether significant subnutrition, malabsorption or bleeding is present.

Some would regard three negative tests for stool occult-blood as an indication that occult bleeding is unlikely, and body weight, serum albumin and calcium as a useful combination to exclude significant subnutrition. To this may be added a dietary history. When investigating the elderly, remember that peptic ulcers and erosions may be painless.

4. Malabsorption of iron does not occur in isolation. The serum folate is often low as well. Combined Fe and folate/B_{12} deficiency may produce normochromic/normocytic anaemia. However, there seems little indication to measure them here.

5. There is a latent period after starting oral iron before a haematological response occurs, but after a week, one might expect a rise of 0.2 g/dl/day. Thus, this lady's Hb would take a month to reach 10 g/dl. This would be no quicker after parenteral therapy.

Question C

1. Since there was no direct evidence of occult bleeding, it would have been useful to have known her weight (45 kg) and have a dietary assessment. Subnutrition is increasingly recognised in the over 80s.

2. The following may be responsible for undiagnosed blood loss: colorectal neoplasm missed by barium enema; a bleeding diathesis; angiodysplasia of the colon; bleeding into the urinary or genital tracts unreported by the patient (ensure that the urine has been tested for blood).

3. The elderly may be very disabled by even modest anaemia because of limited cardiorespiratory or cerebral reserve. Transfusion may be justified to counter immediate symptoms or to speed recovery as in this case. Special care should be taken to avoid precipitating heart failure.

4. Side-effects of i.v. iron therapy include arthralgia in patients with rheumatoid arthritis and exacerbation of urinary infection, due to high urine Fe levels. Both these conditions are common in the elderly. An anaphylactic reaction occasionally occurs.

Suggested further reading

Department of Health and Social Security (1979) Nutrition and health in old age. Report on Health Social Services, No. 16. HMSO, London

Hale W E et al (1983) Haematological and biochemical laboratory values in an ambulatory elderly population. Age and Ageing, 12, 275-284

CASE 16

HEMIPLEGIA

HISTORY

A 75-year-old man was taken to hospital as an emergency, and found on examination by the Senior House Officer to have a left hemiplegia. His wife, who accompanied him, was told that he had suffered a stroke, and the patient was admitted to an acute medical ward. He was drowsy, and made inappropriate responses to commands.

Question A

1. Give one mandatory investigation to be done at this stage.

2. List at least three factors which are important in the prognosis after stroke.

3. List the physical signs which help in establishing a vascular pathology for his symptoms.

4. Are you justified in assuming, as a working diagnosis, that he has had a stroke?

5. List three immediate objectives in the management of this patient.

A further interview with his wife revealed that he had become paralysed suddenly while watching TV and had gradually become more drowsy over a period of 3 hours. There was no history of head trauma. He was not hypertensive but smoked "a few cigarettes a day". Re-examination the next day showed a grade 2/5 flaccid weakness in the left arm and leg. There was marked sensory and visual inattention. His speech was very slurred, but his cough reflex was intact and his swallowing difficult but adequate. He was incontinent of urine and faeces.

Question B

Which of the following statements are true?

1. Hypertensives with strokes do better than non-hypertensives.

2. Infarcts in the dominant hemisphere are worse than those in the non-dominant hemisphere.

3. "Young strokes" do better than "old strokes".

4. The outcome after a stroke can be assessed at the outset.

5. He should be catheterised to protect his pressure areas.

Question C

List three activities of daily living with which this man is likely to have problems, and give the reasons why.

The patient was transferred to the stroke unit in the department of geriatric medicine. His left leg was noted to be swollen but the tone was returning, and the power was 2-3/5. He was still incontinent of urine and faeces. He complained of pain in his left shoulder and also of colicky abdominal pain.

Question D

Discuss:

1.   Why are legs commonly swollen after a stroke?

2.   What is the cause of his painful shoulder, and what should be done about it?

3.   How should the incontinence be treated?

4.   What objectives should be set for him now?

5.   What further information is needed now?

A Doppler ultrasound did not indicate thrombosis in a thigh vein; he was given an anti-embolism stocking, the oedema subsided, and subsequent Doppler ultrasound examinations were also negative. His incontinence was controlled by regular tioletting, and although his shoulder pain improved, he still required analgesics.

After a further 8 weeks he was able to transfer himself from bed to chair unaided, and take a few paces by himself, though insecurely. He could manipulate his wheelchair in the ward. He could dress himself, although he still had a tendency to put his clothes on the wrong way round or inside out. It was decided to send him home in a wheelchair, and continue his rehabilitation as an outpatient in the Day Hospital. A home visit was planned with the physiotherapist and occupational therapist. His wife described the home where they had lived for 40 years as being semidetached, having three bedrooms with a bathroom/lavatory upstairs, and a small, recently-installed lavatory downstairs with two other rooms and a kitchen. She herself was 78 years old, suffered with arthritis of the knees, and used a walking stick.

Question E

List at least three problems you might anticipate on this home visit.

There were several steps up to the house, and a narrow path, so it would not be possible for him to go out in a wheelchair. A nephew was also present for the visit, and brought a divan bed downstairs. The patient was quite unable to rise from this, or from his favourite easy chair. Access to the downstairs toilet was impossible from the wheelchair, although he could move the wheelchair in the house satisfactorily. He was, however, unable to walk over the carpets because of dragging the left foot, and transfers were difficult on this surface.

Question F

Suggest solutions to each of the above five problems.

With the therapists' recommendations implemented and a home-help requested, the patient was sent home. He made good physical progress with further outpatient rehabilitation. However, it soon became apparent that there was a great discrepancy between his performance at hospital and at home. He demanded that his wife dress him and help him on every occasion he wished to move. He took no interest in his old pursuits or in television, and even ignored their few visitors. He was also argumentative, and his wife was finding him impossible to live with. She requested his readmission to hospital.

Question G

How would you tackle this problem?

ANSWERS

Question A

1. The blood sugar should certainly be measured; hypoglycaemia may produce focal neurological signs, particularly in the elderly. The haemoglobin might also be measured to pick up unlikely to change acute management, as might a chest radiograph to help exclude metastatic neoplasia. A clear history and physical examination of the head might be more useful than a skull radiograph.

2. Conscious level; the degree of weakness; and signs of diffuse neurological damage, e.g. gaze palsy, hemianopia and severe sensory disturbance.

3. There are no physical signs which can prove that a patient has suffered a cerebrovascular event, with the possible exception of subhyloid haemorrhage in the retina. The diagnosis must rest on the history and/or specific investigations (e.g. a CT head scan). Some constellations of signs suggest that a particular vascular territory has been affected, but all can be mimicked by other intracranial pathology, e.g. a lateral medullary syndrome; brain stem signs plus central visual field defects; marked differences between the spasticity of the arm

and leg with a significant hemiplegia. Associated signs of hypertension and vascular disease (e.g. bruits) are contributory, but not diagnostic.

4. No, a history has not yet been obtained and therefore an adequate diagnosis cannot be made.

5. Maintenance of an adequate airway, prevention of pressure sores, and adequate hydration.

Question B   1 is correct.

Hypertensives frequently have small "lacunar" strokes affecting the internal capsule. The effects may be severe at the outset, but recovery can be very quick. Patients with no risk-factors are more likely to have suffered a major cerebral infarction and do poorly. Thus, hypertensives are more likely to suffer a stroke, but the outlook for an individual stroke may be relatively good.

There is no clear evidence that the side of a stroke is important in prognosis. There is a suggestion that patients with non-dominant strokes are more difficult to rehabilitate rather than the other way round.

The effect of age on rehabilitation after a stroke is small compared with the effect of the degree of cerebral damage sustained. If age is related, it is probably because of other disabilities present before the stroke, rather than age itself being a factor.

In group analysis, accurate predictions of outcome may be made at the outset of a stroke. For individuals, however, progress may be very variable, and an open mind should be kept for at least a month.

He should be offered a bottle regularly and may well indicate the need to pass water if handled sympathetically. In any event, a sheath would be preferable to a urethral catheter.

Question C

1. Feeding, because visual inattention may lead to him ignoring some of his food.

2. Dressing, because visuo-spacial disorientation is likely with this type of cortical defect.

3. Mobility, because, apart from his weakness, he is flaccid, and is likely to ignore his left leg.

Question D

1. The usual cause for a swollen leg after a stroke is a deep venous thrombosis, which occurs in up to 75%, a third of which may be clots of a significant size.

2. He is likely to have an inflamed joint capsule, or to have subluxed joints through his arm dangling by his side. It should

always be well supported, and often a figure-of-eight strapping is helpful. Care should be taken when moving such patients not to pull on the paralysed arm.

3. He should have a rectal examination to detect faecal impaction, which is very likely, and probably the cause of the abdominal pain. The bowel should then be cleared by regular daily enemas until there is no return, followed by a regular laxative. He should be encouraged to use the urine bottle two hourly, and a chart of his incontinence kept.

4. The major objective must be to get him mobile or at least independent in a wheelchair with the ability to transfer. He also needs to learn to dress, and manage personal hygiene. He should be seen daily by an occupational therapist for this retraining, as well as a physiotherapist.

5. His home and social circumstances need investigation with emphasis on:

    (a) The home layout with reference to future discharge,

    (b) The degree of support at home,

    (c) His previous social activities and hobbies so that appropriate help may be given (e.g. to a keen gardener).

Question E

1. Step up to the house, obstacle to wheelchair.

2. Difficult access to the downstairs toilet.

3. No provision has been made to assess him on a bed.

4. Too many obstacles in the house for his wheelchair.

5. Unsuitable chairs.

Question F

1. Access to the house is likely to remain a problem, even if his mobility improved further.

2. The bed is too low and should be raised with blocks to a suitable height.

3. The easy chair is probably too low, and too backward-slanting. An upright alternative of the right height with arm rests should be found.

4. A commode or chair toilet should be provided unless rails by the downstairs toilet would obviously help.

5. He probably has a foot drop which may make moving on carpets difficult. The carpets, or rugs, could either be removed in key areas or the patient tried with an ankle splint.

Question G

This is a very common scenario after a disabling illness such as stroke and there may be many related factors. Firstly, the patient may be depressed. Secondly, the wife may be over-protective and anxious, not realising his degree of independence. She may benefit from seeing him perform in hospital with the therapists. Thirdly, she may simply be tired of limited social contact.

The patient was started on an antidepressant. His wife was encouraged to go out when he was attending the Day Hospital. They were referred to a Stroke Club (run by the Chest, Heart and Stroke Association), where they could meet others in the same circumstances and discuss problems. They were offered relief admissions to hospital so that she could take a break but they declined this and a volunteer visitor arranged for them to take a holiday-for-the-disabled together. A year later the situation was stable, and the patient was reasonably mobile in the house. He could also get out into his small back garden.

Suggested further reading

Andrews K, Stewart J (1979) Stroke recovery: he can but does he? Rheumatology and Rehabilitation, 18, 43-48

Andrews K et al (1981) The rate of recovery from stroke and its measurement. International Rehabilitation Medicine, 3, 155-161

Mulley G P (1985) Practical Management of Stroke. Croom Helm, London and Sydney

CASE 17

CONFUSION, COUGH
AND AN INFECTED FOOT

HISTORY AND EXAMINATION

An 85-year-old man was admitted from home, acutely ill with fever, cough and dyspnoea. On examination he was thin and was noted to have an infection in the plantar space of the left foot. The foot was hot and otherwise in a healthy condition, as was the right foot. He was disorientated in time and place and resented being examined. There were no abnormal physical signs in the chest but the respiratory rate was 28 per minute, and he was expectorating yellow sputum. Blood pressure 80/50 mmHg. Pulse 120/minute and no signs of heart failure. Fundoscopy was normal.

Ten years previously he had a partial gastrectomy for a peptic ulcer. He had not consulted his general practitioner for some time. He was believed to be only an occasional drinker.

Question A

Which of the following statements are true?

1. Lobar pneumonia is an unlikely diagnosis here.

2. Physical signs are commonly absent in elderly patients with lobar pneumonia.

3. Blood cultures are only rarely positive in the elderly with pneumonia.

4. His urine should be tested for sugar.

5. His foot infection should be allowed to drain spontaneously as in such an elderly patient surgery is likely to lead to amputation.

A chest radiograph showed shadowing in the right mid-zone consistent with lobar consolidation of the right middle lobe. Critical re-examination of the patient showed reduced movements on the right side and a patch of bronchial breathing in the right axilla, which later resolved. Radiographs of the left foot showed no evidence of gas or osteomyelitis. His urine was negative for sugar but the blood glucose was 16 mmol/l. The knee jerks were brisk but it was not possible to test the ankle jerks adequately, the plantar responses were unreactive and he seemed insensitive to pin-prick on the feet, but not on the thighs. Peripheral pulses were all present. Other preliminary investigations showed: Hb 8.6 g/dl; blood urea 15 mmol/l; serum albumin 30 g/l. Blood and urine cultures were taken and the foot wound swabbed; a penicillin-sensitive Staphylococcus was cultured from the foot.

He was treated with intravenous fluids and benzyl penicillin and initially improved.

Question B

Which of the following tests would you prefer to perform to establish the cause of the foot ulcer?

1. Glucose tolerance test

2. Mean corpuscular volume

3. Arteriography of the legs

4. Examination of his shoes

5. Serum zinc

PROGRESS

Despite surgical drainage of his foot and appropriate antibiotics, he developed a rapidly spreading gangrene of the left leg and required a left mid-thigh amputation. Serum B_{12} was less than 50 mg/l and the bone marrow was floridly megaloblastic. He was transfused perioperatively. The blood glucose remained elevated and he was temporarily given insulin, but after surgery the diabetes was controlled by diet alone.

He remained weak and was unable to manage a prosthesis and was later discharged to a nursing home in the community taking monthly vitamin B_{12} (by injection) and a 120 g carbohydrate diet. His sensorimotor neuropathy did not improve, and he was wheelchair-bound. Three months later he was readmitted because he had been persistently incontinent of faeces for 6 weeks and had diarrhoea for which he had been prescribed codeine phosphate.

Question C

Which of the following do you think will be of most value in managing his diarrhoea?

1. Stool culture and microscopy

2. Plain abdominal radiograph

3. Digital examination of the rectum

4. Therapeutic trial of tetracycline

5. Increase the dose of codeine phosphate

Question D

Which one of the following do you think is the disorder most likely to be a complication in this case?

1. Background diabetic retinopathy

2. Sacral pressure sore

3. Ischaemic colitis

4. Hyperuricaemia

5. Pelvic abscess from diverticular disease

Rectal examination revealed gross faecal impaction which responded to withdrawal of codeine, daily enemas and a stimulant laxative. He also had a small sacral pressure sore which healed with the provision of an adequate cushion for the wheelchair, and regular turning while in bed. After these measures his bowels ceased to be a problem. He remained well until a carcinoma of the lung was diagnosed several years later.

ANSWERS

Question A   4

Lobar pneumonia should be considered because he is pyrexial, has a productive cough and is tachypnoeic. Physical signs of a chest infection may genuinely be absent, but it is more common for them to be missed, particularly if the axillae are not examined. Blood cultures are positive in about 20-30% of elderly patients with clear-cut chest infections before antibiotics are given, and should always be taken. Testing the urine for sugar is clearly mandatory; however, because of a higher renal threshold for glucose in the elderly, minor levels of hyperglycaemia may be missed unless the blood is examined also. It is important to allow free drainage of such neuropathic ulcers, by surgery if necessary. The blood supply to the foot is good so there is no contraindication.

Question B   2 and 4

He evidently had diabetes on admission and a GTT would not be helpful at this stage. If doubt about the diagnosis exists later, another random sugar should be measured. The morphology of any anaemia should be assessed. In this case the MCV was 110 fl, which led to the diagnosis of severe vitamin B_{12} deficiency. The integrity of the blood supply to the foot is not in doubt and zinc deficiency is not a factor in this type of ulcer. Neuropathic foot ulcers may be precipitated by ill-fitting shoes or a nail penetrating the sole.

Question C 3

Digital examination of the rectum is mandatory in any elderly patient with diarrhoea or faecal incontinence to exclude impaction.

Infectious diarrhoea is usually obvious from the history. A plain abdominal film may reveal proximal impaction which might otherwise be missed in an obese subject; it is no substitute for rectal examination. Tetracyclines may be useful in neuropathic diarrhoea and in occasional patients with bacterial overgrowth. In patients with neurological incontinence, high doses of constipating agents may be needed but these may cause sedation and confusion in the old.

Question D 2

Background retinopathy is unlikely to have developed over a few months. A sacral pressure sore is likely since he is immobile and faecally incontinent. This should be specifically looked for, and preventative measures undertaken even if the skin had been intact in this case. The other options are possibilities, but not likely in this case.

Suggested further reading

Davidson M B (1970) The effect of aging on carbohydrate metabolism. A review of the English literature and a practical approach to the diagnosis of diabetes mellitus in the elderly. Metabolism, 28, 688-705

Fitzgerald M G, Kilvert A (1985) The endocrine system - diabetes. In: Brocklehurst J C (ed.) Textbook of Geriatric Medicine and Gerontology, 3rd Edn. Churchill Livingstone, Edinburgh

CASE 18

FALLS – 2

HISTORY

An 82-year-old widow was admitted after a fall at home. She had been watching the midnight movie on the television and had fallen from her chair, was unable to get up, and so slept on the floor until morning when she walked to the telephone and summoned help. She has been living on her own in two rooms downstairs for several years. Three years previously she had been admitted after a blackout, was found to be in mild congestive cardiac failure, and was prescribed digoxin and a diuretic. Twenty-four hour ECG monitoring has shown ventricular ectopic beats and second degree heart block with Wenckebach's phenomenon at night. She also had a 20-year history of angina pectoris.

Question A

What significance do you attach to her having spent all night on the floor yet being able to rise and get help the next morning?

ON EXAMINATION

Examination revealed a thin but sprightly lady with an obvious fracture of the left clavicle but no other abnormal physical signs. In particular, examination of the nervous system was normal; pulse 60/minute, regular. Blood pressure 150/85 mmHg. During the physical examination she complained of high back pain which was poorly localised.

Question B

Which of the following are true about heart block?

1. It can be responsible for falls.

2. If a standard (12-lead) ECG does not show periods of asystole, Stokes-Adams attacks are unlikely.

3. A history of loss of consciousness is mandatory for the diagnosis of Stokes-Adams attack.

4. Digoxin is safe to use in the presence of atrioventricular block.

5. It is not worth treating in patients of over 80 years of age.

INVESTIGATIONS

An ECG showed sinus rhythm with no definite abnormality; chest radiograph showed slight cardiomegaly and comminuted fractures of the left clavicle; cervical spine radiograph revealed a fracture through the base of the odontoid peg. She was treated with a collar and cuff and a firm cervical collar. Further investigations showed an Hb 13.4 g/dl, MCV 102 fl, serum B_{12} 295 ng/l, serum folate 3.6 µg/l, CPK 521 iu/l and LDH 504 iu/l.

Question C

Which of the following are true?

1. She is likely to have had a myocardial infarction.

2. Heart block has been excluded as the cause for her fall.

3. There is enough evidence to justify repeating the B_{12} and folate estimations as these are probably wrong.

4. The fractured odontoid peg is likely to be old and unrelated to her present injury.

5. The physical examination was inadequate because the blood pressure was not also measured with the patient standing.

MANAGEMENT

Further enquiry revealed that she drank 3 litres of sherry per week, preferring draught to regular bottled drink because of "trouble getting rid of the empties". On the night in question, she had drunk "several glasses" and slept soundly (and pain-free) on the floor, being able to rise without difficulty in the morning. Twenty-four hour ECG monitoring was normal, and she was discharged after a short stay in hospital, taking frusemide, spironolactone and glyceryl trinitrate.

Question D

What other injuries might she have suffered?

Question E

Which of the following are true?

1. The old generally tolerate alcohol less well than the young.

2. Heavy drinking can be ruled out by a clear history from the patient and measurement of the serum GGT.

3. A confused elderly subject should not be denied a moderate amount of regular alcohol if he has been used to it for a number of years.

4.   Alcoholics are more prone to subdural haematomata.

5.   Alcohol abuse may result in characteristic neuropathological changes, distinct from senile dementia.

ANSWERS

Question A

Spending the night on the floor is not uncommon after a fall; however, the patient usually tries to recover and summon help. After a drop-attack, the subject may be unable to rise for some time but later can walk quite well, and consciousness is not lost. Alternatives are that she had been unconscious (though unaware of this), or sedated.

Question B   1 and 2

Strictly speaking, loss of consciousness must occur for the diagnosis of a Stokes-Adams attack. However, intermittent heart block may be responsible for falls in the absence of a clear history of loss of consciousness or of atrioventricular disassociation on the ECG. The key to the correct diagnosis of any dysrhythmia is finding the abnormality by ECG monitoring and relating it to the patient's symptoms. With heart block, however, a suggestive history and suggestive ECG finding (e.g. trifascicular block) may in themselves be sufficient indications for a pacemaker. The role of digoxin in chronic heart failure is disputed, and in the presence of atrioventricular block, it should be used with great caution. The treatment of heart block with a permanent cardiac pacemaker is worthwhile for the patient even in extreme old age, and, since it often helps the patient to remain out of hospital, treatment with a pacemaker is likely to be cost-effective.

Question C   5

Raised enzymes (CPK and LDH) may occur after a fall and are thus commonly elevated in elderly in-patients. A single intramuscular injection, or a stroke can also raise the CPK to high levels (>1000 iu/l). There is no direct evidence that she suffered a myocardial infarction, though this is by no means ruled out. Likewise, heart block has not been wholly excluded, particularly in view of her history. The finding of a high MCV with normal B_{12} and folate levels should point to the possibility of alcohol excess, liver disease, reticulocytosis or vitamin C deficiency. It is rash to assume that the odontoid peg fracture is old; trauma is generally underestimated in the elderly either because of confusion or, as in this case, because of analgesia and sedation from drugs. We regard the measurement of standing blood pressure as part of the normal physical examination of all older patients, particularly if they have fallen shortly after standing up.

Question D

Rib fractures (often multiple) are common in elderly fallers and alcoholics.

Question E   1, 4 and 5

The old do not tolerate alcohol better than the young but may, for several reasons, be able to hide its effect. The history from the patient (particularly a female) cannot rule out alcohol abuse and under these circumstances an interview with the family and friends, or a domiciliary visit, can be invaluable. The GGT, if raised, may fall after only a few days of abstinence. Even small amounts of alcohol may be deleterious to an already handicapped subject, and thus may have to be banned. Alcoholics, and those with cortical atrophy, seem particularly prone to the development of subdural haematomata. The pathology of senile dementia is that of Alzheimer's disease; alcoholic-associated encephalopathy may result as symmetrical atrophy in the thalamus, hypothalamus, midbrain and mammillary bodies.

Suggested further reading

Caird F I et al (1974) Significance of abnormalities of the electrocardiogram in old age. British Heart Journal, 36, 1012-1018

Caird F I, Dall J L C, Kennedy (eds.) (1976) Cardiology in Old Age. Plenum Press, New York and London

CASE 19

ANTICOAGULANTS
AND PAINFUL KNEES

HISTORY

Mrs M was 66 years old when she first presented with shortness of breath on exertion. She was found, on examination, to have mitral stenosis and incompetence and to be in atrial fibrillation. She did not give a history of rheumatic fever, and seemed fit in other respects. She was prescribed a small dose of a thiazide diuretic, digoxin, 0.25 mg daily, and nicoumalone (a short-acting coumarin-type anticoagulant). The latter was intended to protect against the possible risk of systemic emboli from the left atrium. Her symptoms were markedly improved, and she diligently attended the local Anticoagulant Clinic; her anticoagulant control was considered good.

About 10 years later she began to complain of pain in her knees. She was now living on her own, and her daughter found her increasingly forgetful and less fastidious in looking after herself. Her general practitioner diagnosed osteoarthritis of the knees and started her on regular paracetamol. This gave some relief, but she was still bothered with pain, so he prescribed a non-steroidal anti-inflammatory drug (NSAID) in its place.

Question A

List at least three reasons why anticoagulant treatment in this patient is now more hazardous.

The Anticoagulant Clinic was consulted about this change in therapy, and the patient promptly seen for review; there was no change in her anticoagulant control. The patient continued to become generally more frail, but maintained her independence. Nine months later she became ill, passed melaena and was admitted to hospital as an emergency. Upon admission the haemoglobin was 6.8 g/dl and the prothrombin ratio (British Comparative Ratio) was 1.9 to 1. The pulse was 70/minute (atrial fibrillation) and the blood pressure was 160/85 mmHg. The patient was given one unit of fresh frozen plasma, phytomenadione (vitamin K_1), 20 mg intravenously, and four units of blood were transfused over 24 hours. The nicoumalone was stopped, but her other medications were not changed. The day after admission a gastroscopy showed one large gastric ulcer and a smaller one; there was no evidence of bleeding. The NSAID was stopped and she was started on carbenoxolone, 100 mg three times daily.

Question B

Comment on this treatment.

On the morning of the third day she was noted to have a right hemiparesis. A CT head scan showed a large cerebral infarct. Her rehabilitation was hampered by confusion which was very evident after the stroke (mental test score 4/10) and by a recurrence of pain in the knees which was very troublesome at night. The right knee was slightly hot and swollen. A radiograph of the joint showed degenerative changes, particularly of the patello-femoral joint. Paracetamol and dihydrocodeine were given for pain relief with the effect that she became more confused and incontinent of urine (this resolved when the codeine was stopped). The patient became very tearful and refused to put any weight on her right leg. Her urea was 15 mmol/l (her fluid intake was poor) and the ESR was 86 mm/hour.

Question C

Suggest three possible causes of her joint problem, and the diagnostic steps you would take.

Turbid fluid was aspirated from the right knee, and numerous monosodium-urate crystals were seen together with polymorphonuclear leukocytes. The serum uric acid was marginally elevated. She was treated with colchicine with dramatic benefit, and because she needed to continue with a diuretic, allopurinol was later added. The patient did not regain her independence and remained in hospital, comfortable after the above measures.

ANSWERS

Question A

1. There may be an interaction between the non-steroidal anti-inflammatory drug (NSAID) and her anticoagulant. This effect varies widely with different drugs in this class, but, in general, providing the laboratory controlling the anticoagulant is aware of the change, and the drug is taken regularly, this should not create too much of a problem.

2. NSAIDs are also associated with peptic ulcers and there is therefore an increased risk of bleeding. Such ulcers are not uncommonly pain-free in the elderly.

3. She has become more forgetful, and she is now on four drugs (a diuretic, digoxin, nicoumalone and the NSAID); there is therefore the risk that compliance will be poor. Furthermore, she may not report symptoms (such as bruising or bleeding) which might otherwise alert her attendants to the risk of a potentially serious bleed.

4. The arthritis of the knees and her brain failure make her more prone to fall, and thus increase the risks associated with anticoagulation. The fact that she lives alone is a further hazard.

Question B

The patient had almost certainly been bleeding from her peptic ulcer(s), but this may have been fairly slow, because her pulse and blood pressure were not seriously deranged, the haemoglobin was low on admission, and she had passed melaena rather than vomited blood. It was, however, certainly wise to transfuse her to a safer level. The prothrombin time was not excessively prolonged, and the anticoagulant was probably a contributory factor to the bleeding, rather than the prime cause. Fresh frozen plasma would have been adequate to reverse the minor clotting abnormality present and the dose of vitamin K given was too large. Transfusion of the elderly, particularly those known to have impaired cardiac function, should be monitored closely to avoid pulmonary oedema. Central venous pressure measurements may be very helpful though are often neglected in this age group.

After gastrointestinal haemorrhage, the elderly more commonly bleed again and require surgery than the young, so it is customary in many units for physicians to liaise with a surgeon from the time of admission. The prescription of carbenoxolone is unjustified owing to its fluid-retaining properties (it is chemically similar to aldosterone). Cimetidine and ranitidine are commonly prescribed in high doses in this situation, but the elderly may become confused on these drugs. The bismuth chelate "De-nol" may be the drug of choice for the elderly, but should only be given in short courses because of the potential toxicity of absorbed bismuth.

Question C

The most fruitful investigation would be a joint aspiration. This might reveal a septic arthritis or a crystal arthropathy, either gout or pseudo-gout. Acute rheumatoid arthritis is also another possibility. If the synovial fluid was not turbid on aspiration, a long-acting steroid and local anaesthetic could be instilled at the same time. This may give great symptomatic relief.

Suggested further reading

Grahame R (1985) The musculoskeletal system - disease of the joints. In: Brocklehurst J C (ed.) Textbook of Geriatric Medicine and Gerontology, 3rd Edn. Churchill Livingstone, Edinburgh

Shepherd A M M et al (1977) Age as a determinant of sensitivity to Warfarin. British Journal of Clinical Pharmacology, 4, 312-320

CASE 20

TERMINAL DISTRESS

CASE I

Mr J had severe emphysema, and had been short of breath for years. When he developed jaundice he was admitted to an acute geriatric assessment ward where a diagnosis of carcinoma of the pancreas was made on the basis of ultrasound and CT evidence of extrahepatic biliary obstruction and a mass in the head of the pancreas. He was not completely obstructed, as shown by moderate urobilinogen in the urine and modest, stable elevation of the serum bilirubin. He was judged unfit for any form of surgery because of poor respiratory reserve. He was losing weight rapidly, could not get out of bed unaided, and was only able to take a few paces. He was also incontinent of urine unless toiletted. Only the patient's wife was told the diagnosis, and she decided to try to nurse him at home. He was therefore discharged on the following day.

Question A

1. On the information given above, are there any points in his management you might criticise?

2. Make a list of the problems that you think this patient might have on discharge.

CASE II

Mr P had been a very active man all his life, having had a long career in the Navy. He suffered an apparently uncomplicated myocardial infarction, but 3 years later he presented in very severe congestive cardiac failure. He was treated with diuretics and later a vasodilator and discharged, but after a short period he had to be readmitted. He was then described as being in very severe congestive cardiac failure and extremely short of breath. He was told that the prognosis was very poor. He refused to eat, continually said that he wished to die, and later tried to commit suicide by strangling himself with the tube to his oxygen mask.

Question B

1. What factors might be related to his suicidal behaviour?

2. Give a simple account of how you might manage this man.

CASE III

Mrs B had suffered from rheumatoid arthritis for many years and had been treated with oral corticosteroids. She had unfortunately become quite cushingoid and had crush fractures of several vertebral bodies. She then developed chronic renal failure and congestive cardiac failure which was later shown to be due, at least in part, to amyloidosis. One day she fell and fractured her neck of femur, which required surgery. Postoperatively, she developed pneumonia and a pressure sore and became very weak. It was clear that she would never walk again and she was transferred to a long-stay geriatric ward. On transfer, she was depressed and crying. She resented being moved and seemed to be getting considerable pain from her back and from her pressure sore when the dressings were being changed. Her daughter commented that "all the fight seemed to have gone out of her". Prior to this episode she had been a proud, independent old lady of 85 years who lived on her own with almost no help except with the shopping.

Question C

List some of the factors which you think might be contributing to her depression, and how you might deal with them.

CASE IV

Mrs W was 82 when multiple myeloma was diagnosed. She had multiple skeletal deposits, but normal renal function, and seemed to have a good response to cytotoxic agents. However, within 18 months of diagnosis she developed several episodes of pneumonia and urinary tract infection which led to a gradual deterioration in her health, and ultimately renal failure. Her marriage had always been stormy, and her husband had reacted poorly to her failing health and frequent hospital visits and admissions. Their relationship gradually deteriorated with her health, and when she became immobile she had to be admitted for nursing care. She was anaemic (Hb 6.0 g/dl) and in severe back pain. The haematologist who had been looking after her advised that her prognosis was only a few months and that her chemotherapy should be stopped. Mrs W remained lucid and continually enquired about her drug therapy and when she might be discharged.

Question D

List at least two problems and how they may be managed.

CASE V

A family doctor asked the local geriatric unit to admit one of his elderly patients for terminal care. The patient (a man aged 73) had been diagnosed as suffering from carcinoma of the bronchus 1 year previously and had been getting progressively weaker and had recently refused all food. His wife said that she could no longer cope. Since the unit was full, the matter was referred to the consultant who elected to do a domiciliary assessment. On arrival at the house, he was met by the wife and ushered into a private room. She begged that her husband be taken into hospital, and that on no account should he be told that he had cancer. She would not come into the man's bedroom and so the doctor saw the patient alone. He was cachectic, incontinent of urine and somewhat disorientated in time, but otherwise fully rational. He had not eaten for several days. When it was suggested that he should come into hospital, the patient demanded to know why, what treatment he would be given, and how long he would stay there. The consultant's reply with generalities about investigation and treatment was met with more specific questions and objections by the patient. The wife begged that he be removed.

Question E

How would you handle this?

ANSWERS

CASE I

It does not appear that the patient had been consulted before these decisions were made; it is unlikely that someone who has gone yellow, and is losing weight fast will not suspect something serious is wrong. It is not clear whether his wife has been offered any advice on how to manage him at home, and nor has any definite arrangement for review or readmission been put to them.

The immediate problems that he may encounter are: they may need simple advice on the type of food he might manage, or on the use of anti-nausea drugs. He is likely to have difficulty using the toilet; a bottle urinal and possibly a commode should have been provided. They will need a supply of incontinence pads, and possibly help from the laundry service.

In the longer term, he may become itchy, confused and is likely to develop back pain, all of which will need the intervention of a sympathetic family doctor. If he becomes completely immobile his wife may have great difficulty dealing with him, and the question of increased home nursing, a hospice or readmission to hospital may have to be considered.

CASE II

Apart from endogenous depression, much the most likely cause for his distress would be his physical condition. He was severely hypoxic, continually short of breath and frightened to lie down. He was treated with oxygen, chlorpromazine and morphine and was calm within 24 hours. He died 3 days later.

CASE III

She might be depressed because of the pain, continued activity of her rheumatoid disease, and the loss of her independence. Someone who has non-malignant disease may be in just as much pain as a person with cancer and adequate analgesia should not be withheld just because a condition does not seem "terminal". She was given a small dose of morphine intramuscularly 1 hour before her dressings with great benefit. Her joints continued to be painful, and the corticosteroids were increased slightly, and regular simple analgesia added. In addition, a sedative tricyclic antidepressant was given at night. After 4 weeks her pressure sore was healing well, the morphine was withdrawn, and she was able to sit up and take an interest in the activities around the ward. She no longer cried, and no longer complained of pain. She died some months later of pneumonia.

CASE IV

Some of her problems are:

1. Anaemia. Even terminally ill patients may feel better if their anaemia is corrected. In this case the severe anaemia was due to marrow infiltration. She was transfused to an Hb of 14 g/dl with good effect. She was transfused again twice in the 4 months after this.

2. Back pain. Her back pain could be treated with analgesics, or it might respond to radiotherapy. In this case she was adamant that she did not want to take sedating drugs, and a course of spinal irradiation was arranged. After 4 weeks her back pain was much improved, and controlled with aspirin, 900 mg 3 times daily.

3. Family problems. Her relationship with her husband was obviously distressing her. He was interviewed by both the medical and social work staff, and the terminal nature of his wife's illness emphasised. When a clear idea of the prognosis was understood by him, he agreed to take her home, with regular admissions to hospital (two weeks in and four weeks out). This continued for 7 months until she was admitted for her final illness.

CASE V

It is clear that this couple were not able to discuss his illness. He was close to death, and it seems unlikely that many people reach this stage without realising they are seriously ill; the diagnosis had never been discussed with him. It would also be very difficult to remove him to hospital against his will in these circumstances.

Despite his wife's protestations, the patient was told that he was seriously ill, he remarked that he thought he had cancer, and this was confirmed. He also said that he had a pact with his wife that neither would let the other die in hospital (she confirmed this). After discussing the matter openly for a time, a plan was agreed. The district nurses were to provide incontinence pads for the bed, and a night nurse was arranged through the Marie Curie Foundations (or the Macmillan Nurses in other areas). A small dose of morphine and chlorpromazine was prescribed. He died peacefully 4 days later. The geriatrician subsequently received a letter thanking him for bringing the matter into the open; the wife had had a hard time nursing her husband in those 4 days, but in retrospect was very glad he had not been admitted. It is unlikely that he would have died peacefully if he had been admitted against his will.

Suggested further reading

Brocklehurst J C, Allen S C (1986) Care of the dying. In: Geriatric Medicine for Students, 3rd Edn. Churchill Livingstone, Edinburgh

Hinton J (1972) Dying. Penguin, Harmondsworth

Kubler-Ross E (1970) On Death and Dying. Tavistock Publications, London

CASE 21

ANAEMIA - 2

HISTORY

A 78-year-old lady was seen in the outpatient follow-up clinic. She had been recently discharged from hospital, where she had been investigated for a haematemesis, found at gastroscopy to have a shallow gastric ulcer and treated with a blood transfusion and cimetidine. She had been taking ibuprofen, which was stopped as it was thought to have probably contributed to the formation of the ulcer.

During the 6 weeks between discharge from hospital and the outpatient review, her haemoglobin had fallen from 11.0 g/dl to 8.4 g/dl, though she had had no further haematemesis or melaena.

She was readmitted to hospital for investigations, the results of which were as follows:

Hb 8.4 g/dl, normochromic, normocytic film, reticulocytes < 1%,
WCC 6.5, normal differential

Faecal occult blood negative x 4

Serum iron, TIBC, red cell folate and serum B_{12} all normal

ESR 105 mm/hour

Gastroscopy - the ulcer had healed completely

Question A

True or false?

This patient's anaemia:

1. Is probably due to further upper gastrointestinal bleeding.

2. Is probably due to chronic blood loss from another site.

3. Could be drug-induced.

4. Is not unusual in an old person after an upper gastrointestinal bleed.

5. Could be due to bone marrow infiltration.

Further investigations were as follows:

Blood urea 30.1 mmol/l
Serum albumin 28 g/l
Total protein 78 g/l
Serum calcium 2.20 mmol/l
Alkaline phosphatase 25 iu/l

Question B

In view of these indices, which of the following is most likely to give a diagnostic result?

1. Creatinine clearance estimation.

2. Direct and indirect Coomb's tests.

3. Plasma protein electrophoresis.

4. Serum parathyroid hormone assay.

5. A liver biopsy.

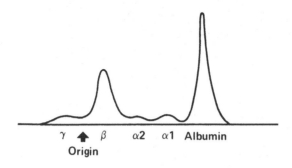

Figure 12 Plasma protein electrophoresis

Question C

What is the abnormality on the plasma protein electrophoresis tracing in Figure 12? How could you confirm which type of abnormal protein is present?

Question D

Describe three other investigations which can yield useful information in patients suspected of having myeloma.

Question E

Describe the various pathological forms which myelomas can adopt.

Question F

Which of the following can be indications for chemotherapy in patients with myeloma?

1. Bence-Jones proteinuria greater than 1 g/24 h

2. Falling haemoglobin

3. Plasmacytoma with normal plasma proteins

4.   A blood urea of 15 mmol/l or more

5.   Bone pain

Question G

Describe treatment, other than chemotherapy, for the following complications of myeloma:

1.   Severe pain from a mid-shaft femoral deposit.

2.   Acute retinal artery occlusion.

3.   Sudden worsening of renal failure.

4.   Acute gout in a metatarsophalangeal joint.

5.   Spinal cord compression.

Question H

True or false?

Bence-Jones proteins in the urine:

1.   Are often accompanied by albuminuria.

2.   Are pathognomic of myeloma.

3.   Consist of kappa and lambda light chains in approximately equal proportions in most cases.

4.   Are proportionally related to prognosis.

5.   Can be present when plasma protein electrophoresis is normal.

ANSWERS

Question A   3 and 5 are true.

Aplastic or hypoplastic anaemias caused by drug toxicity or idiosyncracy could lead to the clinical and haematological picture seen in this case, though these have not been reported in association with cimetidine or ibuprofen. Of course, patients have quite frequently been taking other medications, unknown to their physicians. A drug-related haemolytic anaemia is unlikely in this case, since the reticulocyte count is low.

There are a number of features which point toward bone marrow infiltration; these are the low haemoglobin and reticulocyte count despite normal iron, folate and vitamin B_{12} levels, the absence of evidence of bleeding and the high ESR, though these are not firmly diagnostic of marrow infiltration. Negative faecal occult blood tests do not rule out gastrointestinal bleeding entirely, but in the presence of a normal serum iron and reticulocyte count, and when the ulcer has healed, it becomes unlikely. Similarly, if blood was being lost chronically from another site, such as the urinary tract, the anaemia would usually be hypochromic and microcytic and the serum iron low. In the absence of further bleeding and when iron stores are adequate, the haemoglobin should rise to the normal range within six weeks, even in old age.

Question B   3

The total protein is markedly raised, though the albumin is low. Plasma protein electrophoresis can detect which proteins are abnormally raised, and in view of the renal failure, and raised serum calcium (corrected for the low albumin) despite a normal alkaline phosphatase, it is necessary to look for the monoclonal electrophoretic band which is usually present in multiple myeloma. Creatinine clearance estimation would only quantify the degree of renal failure, not diagnose its cause. Since haemolysis is very unlikely in this patient, the Coomb's tests will not help. The high serum calicum is more likely to be due to myeloma than hyperparathyroidism in view of the high total protein and the normal alkaline phosphatase. There are no firm indications for performing a liver biopsy at this stage.

Question C

The tracing shows an abnormally tall peak in the β-globulin region; this is usually due to a gross excess of a single protein in the IgA class, though IgG, IgM and IgA monoclonal bands are usually in the γ-region. IgD myelomas cause less distinct electrophoretic patterns. The abnormal protein can be further characterised by immunoelectrophoresis.

Question D

1. Qualitative and quantitative testing for Bence-Jones protein in the urine. These consist of light chains and are most commonly caused by myeloma.

2. Bone marrow examination often reveals infiltration with plasmacytes; this is often intense when the peripheral blood indices suggest marrow suppression. The presence of excessive plasmacytes in bone marrow is not absolutely diagnostic of myeloma, as it can occur in other conditions such as chronic infection, chronic liver disease and "collagen" diseases.

3. A skeletal radiological survey helps to determine the extent of the disease, and the presence of multiple lytic bone lesions or vertebral crush fractures is a strong indication to begin chemotherapy.

Question E

Myelomata can secrete protein of any one of the immunoglobulin heavy chain classes (IgG, IgM, IgA, IgD or IgE) in addition to light chains. They can present in various pathological forms:

1. Multiple myeloma. The commonest form, in which malignant plasma cells are disseminated, largely in bone marrow. This is common in the elderly and is slightly more frequent in men.

2. Localised myeloma. One or two plasma cell tumours are present without generalised dissemination of malignant plasma cells. These are sometimes called plasmacytomas. About 50% show a low level monoclonal band on electrophoresis. The patients must be followed up carefully to detect a transformation to multiple myeloma.

3. Indolent myeloma. This is a term applied to low grade myelomata which are asymptomatic and discovered on routine biochemical testing. Though treatment is not needed at this stage, the patients should be seen regularly as a proportion of these myelomata become overt multiple myelomata and may require chemotherapy.

Question F   1, 2, 4 and 5

The aim of chemotherapy in myeloma is to reduce or prevent disability and complications; it is probably very rarely curative. Chemotherapy for myeloma has become a very specialised field, and should be supervised by an oncologist or clinical haematologist. Heavy Bence-Jones proteinuria can lead to accelerated renal damage and should therefore be reduced by chemotherapy in order to keep severe renal failure at bay for as long as possible. When plasma cell infiltration in the bone marrow is intense, red blood cell production is impaired and the patient becomes progressively anaemic; chemotherapy will often lead to a rise in haemoglobin. Renal failure signifies a poor prognosis and should be regarded as an indication for chemotherapy; when renal failure is severe, the prognosis is very poor regardless of the treatment regimen. Bone pain sometimes improves after chemotherapy.

Question G

1. Localised bone pain which is not relieved by chemotherapy or analgesics will often respond to radiotherapy.

2. Plasma viscosity is high and sludging can occur in small vessels; this is probably more common in patients with IgM myelomata, and is more likely to occur when large amounts of the abnormal protein are present. Plasmaphoresis quickly reduces the protein levels and improves small vessel perfusion. The main aim is to prevent occlusion of the retinal artery in the other eye, though the affected eye may improve.

116

Chemotherapy, to reduce malignant plasma cell mass, should be given also.

3. If renal failure worsens abruptly care should be taken to ensure adequate hydration in order to reduce the risk of protein coagulation in renal tubules. Infection, such as septicaemia or ascending urinary infection, should be sought and treated vigorously. Blood pressure must be maintained. In severe cases dialysis is needed, sometimes combined with plasmaphoresis, while chemotherapy is given. It is advisable to seek the advice of a nephrologist under these circumstances; the prognosis is poor.

4. Hyperuricaemia and gout are common in myeloma sufferers. The pain of an acute attack is best controlled with a non-steroidal anti-inflammatory drug, such as indomethacin. The joint should be rested. Allopurinol lowers serum uric acid and helps prevent further attacks.

   The hyperuricaemia of myeloma is due to increased uric acid production by the high turnover of malignant plasma cells and reduced renal excretion of urate as renal function declines. Plasma cell destruction during chemotherapy can lead to a further rise in serum uric acid.

5. When a myeloma tumour is compressing the spinal cord, radiotherapy is often effective. Decompressive laminectomy is required if radiotherapy does not provide a satisfactory response.

Question H   1, 4 and 5 are true.

The proteinuria of myelomata mainly consists of light chains, though in many patients a mild to moderate degree of albuminuria also occurs. Heavier albuminuria generally heralds a decline in renal function and is an indication for chemotherapy.

Bence-Jones proteinuria is most commonly due to myeloma, but can also be present in patients with primary amyloidosis, and in a small proportion of patients with macroglobulinaemia.

The vast majority of multiple myelomata are truly monoclonal and produce either kappa or lambda light chains, not both.

The quantity of Bence-Jones proteins excreted is a reflection of neoplastic plasma cell mass in most cases; heavy excretion is associated with a poor prognosis, principally because of renal failure, and is an indication for chemotherapy.

In about 20% of patients only abnormal light chains are detectable at the time of diagnosis; such patients will have a light chain peak on urine protein electrophoresis and normal plasma protein electrophoresis.

Suggested further reading

Durie B G M, Salmon S E (1982) The current status and future prospects of treatment for multiple myeloma. Clinics in Haematology, **11**, 181-210

Parker D, Malpas J S (1979) Multiple myeloma. Journal of the Royal College of Physicians (London), **13**, 146-153

CASE 22

OLD AGE ABUSE

CASE I

Mrs B had five children. She ran a guest house, and, when each of her children was about 5 years old, she would send them to her mother to be looked after as she found it too much to see to them and the guests. Her mother, who was about 30 years older, ran another guest house nearby. Mrs B was always very forthright, making it clear what she thought and what she wanted, and her children were similar in this regard. It was said that a normal family conversation would seem like a major row to an outsider, yet all the children remained close and visited their mother regularly. When Mrs B stopped working she took little interest in anything, including her house and appearance. She was always plump, but by the time she was 70 years old she weighed about 20 stones. She suffered increasingly from arthritic pains and went to live with one of her daughters who did everything for her. Ultimately, she developed severe heart and renal failure and was admitted to hospital. She improved with treatment but remained bed-bound and had a urinary catheter for persistent urinary incontinence. The hospital sought to discharge her but her first daughter did not feel that she could cope with her any longer. Since it was thought that her life expectancy was a few weeks or months, her second daughter offered to take her in; she herself was physically disabled. Eighteen months later her mother was still ruling the house from an upstairs bedroom. She was unable to move herself in bed, was demanding, and often woke her daughter at night to get a cup of tea and so on. She remained perfectly alert and had no significant brain failure.

About this time, the daughter sought help from the local geriatric unit, and much against Mrs B's wishes, she was brought into hospital for regular intermittent relief admissions. Although this provided a physical relief for her daughter, the patient's demanding nature was, if anything, made worse by this. A few months later the daughter went to her general practitioner to confess that she had hit her mother once on the face after Mrs B had taken a swipe at her in the middle of the night. The general practitioner wrote to the consultant in charge requesting permanent admission to hospital. His letter stated that mother and daughter always seemed to be verbally abusing each other when he called, and now that things had become physical, it all seemed to have got out of hand.

CASE II

Mr E was 73 when he suffered a myocardial infarction followed by a left hemiplegia. This left him severely disabled; he could dress with help and move slowly in the house with the help of a caliper and frame, though he spent most of his time in a wheelchair. His wife was 17 years younger than him, and they had only been married 6 years before this stroke, both having been married and had children before. Six years later he was referred to outpatients because he had broken his caliper and become immobile and incontinent.

Examination showed him to be withdrawn and apathetic. He had some bruising on his upper arms but no other signs of injury. He maintained that his wife had hit him regularly over the previous few weeks. She denied any problem in their marital relations and explicitly denied any physical violence. The patient was offered admission to hospital for a period of assessment and rehabilitation and accepted this keenly. His wife, however, was adamant that he should not be admitted and persuaded him to refuse.

CASE III

Mr L worked for a medium-sized engineering firm for about 25 years. He never married and lived at home with his mother, to whom he always paid a weekly rent. He suffered from grand mal epilepsy all his life, and this was exacerbated when in his later years he began to drink excessively. Over the latter few years, relations with his mother had become strained and ultimately he was unable to work because of drink, and was drawing sick pay. At the age of 64 years he took a large overdose of his anticonvulsants and was comatose for a week. He had a stormy course on an intensive care unit and required a temporary tracheostomy. Two months after this he was still unable to walk and appeared depressed and withdrawn. He scored normally on a mental status questionnaire. His mother and brother visited him while he was in the intensive care unit, but seldom did so once he was moved to a rehabilitation ward. While Mr L was in ICU, his mother had obtained a proxy such that she could sign for his sick pay etc. Despite many attempts to arrange a meeting, the family did not attend. Finally a solicitor (acting for the mother) contacted the consultant in charge with a view to obtaining a Court of Protection order since the patient was clearly incapable of managing his own financial affairs.

CASE IV

Mrs F had lived on her own since her husband died 7 years before. She had always been an alert active woman who had "kept a good house". Unfortunately, over the last 2 years she had become forgetful and had let things slip a little. For a year she had suffered from recurrent falls and in one of these she had fractured the neck of her right femur and had to be admitted to hospital to have this fixed internally. She was transferred to the geriatric unit afterwards. She was occasionally confused at night but by day scored 8 out of 10 in a mental status test. She was mobilised and was partly independent in dressing, but the occupational therapist found her incapable of making even a cup of tea in the ward kitchen; the reason for this was not obvious. Mrs F's son and daughter lived about 20 miles away, and were very anxious that she be admitted to a local authority elderly persons home. Mrs F, however, was firmly set against this. The family were interviewed by the medical social worker, and after this a letter was received stating that they would regard it as "criminal" to send the old lady home. She was taken to view two homes, but despite this she did not change her mind. Meals-on-wheels could only be organised 5 days per week, and it was considered that she would be unable to dress completely, and unable to prepare anything other than the simplest snack. She was also still subject to falls; she had had two in hospital, and no treatable factor could be found. The family were seen by the senior house officer, and they expressed the view that she should be taken to a residential home for a trial period despite her objection, and repeated their threat to institute legal proceedings should anything "happen" to their mother. The doctor agreed with them.

Question A

List three general ways in which old people may be abused.

Question B

Outline a plan of how you would approach the four cases above, with particular reference to:

1. In Case I, should the consultant comply with the general practitioner's request?

2. Would you categorise Case II as "high risk" or "low risk" for further physical violence?

3. What two basic steps should you take when dealing with a request for a Court of Protection order?

4. In Case IV what further could be done to clarify the position?

ANSWERS

Question A

Vulnerable people may be abused physically, mentally or financially.

1. Physical abuse. This may be related to their own person, or to their environment or property. Examples of this are:

   > Abuse of the person - personal violence, or sexual abuse.

Abuse of property - vandalism, robbery either by family members or others, eviction, locking-out or, conversely, locking-in against their will.

2. Mental abuse. This comprises mental cruelty, persistent harrassment, framing or deliberate social isolation and so on.

3. Financial abuse. This relates to the elderly person's assets. For example, failure to provide facilities, misappropriation of funds, manipulation to prevent reasonable expenditure for the benefit of the abused.

Question B

CASE I

One basic principle in dealing with abuse is that proposed remedies may be less acceptable to the sufferer than continued abuse. Therefore, the GP's request should not be complied with until the patient's views have been sought. The daughter and patient should be interviewed separately and together to try and find their respective views of the situation. Special consideration should be given to evidence of other types of abuse than the one admitted to by the daughter. Specific helpful measures might be: offering more support, particularly domiciliary help, and follow-up counselling by a social worker to help the daughter cope with feelings of guilt.

CASE II

This man is clearly at considerable risk: the physical abuse has been repeated; it is confirmed by a second source; the wife denies abuse; the patient is unhappy and withdrawn. The main aim must be to establish exactly what is happening and his precise level of disability. This might be quickly achieved by admission or alternatively, close outpatient supervision (e.g. in a Day Hospital). In the latter case, close liaison with the family doctor would be essential. An effort should be made to relieve the burden on his wife by improving his independence, increasing domiciliary support or offering relief admissions.

CASE III

When considering an application for a Court of Protection order, the two basic steps which must be taken are: (a) to satisfy yourself that the patient really does need his affairs managing for him, and (b) that the person, or persons instituting this, if appointed trustees, really will act in his best interests (members of the family may not always be suitable for this role). Therefore the following are necessary:

1. Make an assessment of the patient's mental state, including a screening test for chronic brain failure. This patient was considered to be within normal limits.

2.   Assess the extent of his financial affairs. Someone with a complex set of investments would clearly have a different need to someone with just a retirement pension. Remember that many people may have significant mental impairment, but yet be able to clearly indicate their personal preference.

         Mr L, since he is nearing retirement, may have to make important decisions about his occupational pension.

3.   Interview members of the family to learn their attitude. A social worker may help with this.

CASE IV

Do not forget that doctors and other hospital workers can abuse patients by ordering them about against their wishes. Moving such patients against their wishes (when their cerebral function is clearly sufficient for them to make such a decision) would not be lawful. On the other hand, it is the duty of the doctor in charge to ensure that the case has been put to the patient as fairly as possible, including being taken, if necessary, to visit new accommodation. Furthermore, it might be negligent to allow a completely incompetent person to live by themselves. A trial discharge may convince the patient that she can no longer manage, or it may show that the hospital staff were too pessimistic. Some patients perform much better in their own homes than in a strange environment; a home visit with the therapists may pick this up.

OUTCOME

CASE I

It became clear that the daughter felt very guilty about hitting her mother but the latter was quite content to stay with the current arrangements and refused long-term admission. The daughter declined any further help in the home, but the hospital social worker made regular visits to counsel and keep an eye on them. However, after 6 months relations declined further and the patient accepted permanent admission to a long-stay ward.

CASE II

The patient was admitted to a rehabilitation ward. His caliper was repaired and he was mobilised to the extent that he could transfer safely on his own between bed, chair and toilet. He was treated with an antidepressant and as his mood improved, his continence returned. It appeared that his wife had withheld food, thrown a drink at him, and left him alone for long periods. Despite this, it was felt that his behaviour was a response to his increased dependency. Since this had improved, he returned home after 4 weeks and matters remained stable thereafter.

CASE III

It was considered that there were no medical grounds for recommending a Court of Protection order. Further enquiries revealed that there was a considerable "balance" of sick pay left, several bank accounts as well as a long-service lump sum due and an occupational pension. His Union obtained the services of a solicitor to whom he gave power of attorney. After several weeks of negotiations his bank books were acquired, and his pension was taken as a lump sum. He had thus found himself with enough money to maintain himself at the private nursing home of his choice for over 7 years.

CASE IV

After further discussions with the family, the patient's GP, and support services, it was decided to send the patient home. The occupational therapist also checked that there were no obvious modifications required. The patient had meals-on-wheels 5 days weekly and a visitor (including a home-help) daily to leave other food out. Mrs F muddled along better than most had expected; she died 9 months later of a myocardial infarction. She never changed her mind about staying in her own home.

Suggested further reading

Eastman M (1984) Old Age Abuse. Age Concern, England

CASE 23

SWELLING OF A
HEMIPARETIC LEG

CASE I

Mr C was a 76-year-old barrister who collapsed at home while having an after-work drink. He was brought into hospital and found to have a global dysphasia, and a complete paresis of the right side of the body. Inquiry revealed that he had developed congestive cardiac failure about 6 months previously and had been regularly taking a diuretic since. He was incontinent of urine and catheter-ised. Over the next 2 weeks he made no progress, and was referred to a stroke rehabilitation unit. Re-examination at this stage showed a flicker of movement in the right side of his face and at the right shoulder, but no other movements on the right side. His blood pressure was 160/90 mmHg, the left ventricle was clinically enlarged with an apical systolic murmur and a quiet fourth heart sound. There was marked pitting oedema of the right leg, and an area of redness over the buttocks.

CASE II

Mrs F, aged 68 years, was obese and suffered from osteoarthrosis. She fell and fractured the neck of her right femur, for which a metal prosthesis was inserted. Postoperatively, she made good progress and after 10 days she was transferred to an orthopaedic-geriatric rehabilitation unit. At this time she was noted to have gross pitting oedema of the right leg. She was treated with an intravenous infusion of heparin.

Question A

The incidence of detectable DVT after a fracture of the neck of femur in the elderly is approximately:

1.   20%

2.   25%

3.   40%

4.   50%

5.   60%

6.   90%

Question B

The incidence of detectable DVT after an acute hemiplegia in the elderly is approximately:

1. 15%
2. 20%
3. 25%
4. 40%
5. 50%
6. 60%

Question C

Which of the following statements are true?

1. The swelling of Mr C's right leg is highly indicative of DVT.

2. Swelling of a hemiplegic limb is most commonly due to the paresis and local changes in blood flow.

3. Mr C's diuretic dose should be increased because he had signs of worsening cardiac failure.

4. Mrs F should have been investigated for a possible DVT before being anticoagulated.

5. Although DVT is common after both stroke and fractured femur, pulmonary embolism is comparatively rare.

Mr C had a Doppler ultrasound (DU) performed which demonstrated a complete block of his right femoral vein. A significant proximal vein thrombosis was therefore diagnosed and the patient was treated with intravenous heparin and later with an oral anticoagulant. At the same time he wore a graduated-pressure stocking on both legs. In the case of Mrs F, a venogram was normal (including the pelvic veins visualised) and anticoagulants were stopped.

Question D

Which of the following are true of methods of diagnosing a DVT?

1. Venography is the quickest investigation.

2. Venography is the most specific investigation.

3. ^{125}I fibrinogen scanning (IFS) is the most sensitive technique and accurately diagnoses the mildest and most severe DVTs.

4. Impedance plethesmography (IPG) is sensitive for proximal vein thrombosis, but not for calf vein thrombosis.

5. Doppler ultrasound is more sensitive for calf vein thrombosis than the IPG.

Question E

Which of the following statements are true concerning the use of anticoagulants in the elderly?

1.   Heparin (5000 units subcutaneously 12 hourly) offers safe prophylaxis (from DVT) for old patients undergoing elective or emergency hip surgery.

2.   The ageing process makes the old more likely to bleed on oral anticoagulants than the young.

3.   Cardiac failure may be an indication for anticoagulating an immobile patient.

4.   In a patient with a proven DVT, the risks of anticoagulants after a stroke far outweigh any beneficial effect from preventing pulmonary embolism.

5.   Patients who have just undergone hip surgery should be screened for the development of DVT and offered conventional anticoagulant therapy if evidence of a DVT is found.

PROGRESS

Mrs F made an uneventful recovery and continued to live by herself. Mr C was anticoagulated for 3 months without mishap. His recovery from the stroke was limited but he went home after 8 months in hospital.

ANSWERS

Question A   5 is correct.

Question B   4 is correct.

Estimates of the incidence of DVT depend on the methods used for diagnosis, the more sensitive the method, the more DVTs are found. With fractured neck of femur, the incidence of pelvic vein thrombosis is perhaps higher than in stroke, and the thrombosis rate is higher in traumatic rather than elective hip surgery, and also probably higher among older subjects. The total DVT rate in both hip fractures and stroke is in excess of 50%, and in most series up to 75%.

Question C   1 and 4 are correct.

If oedema develops in a limb after a stroke, this is highly suggestive (>80% specific) of a DVT. If oedema extends above the knee and is unilateral, a severe DVT is almost certain. The most common cause of a swollen limb after hemiplegia is a DVT.

No signs of worsening cardiac failure have been mentioned. If his central venous pressure was elevated, a pulmonary embolus

127

might be expected as there is an approximately 50% chance of a clinically detectable embolus when a large proximal vein thrombosis is present.

Oedema of the leg after a hip fracture may be due to the trauma and surgery rather than a DVT.

About 25% of patients with these two conditions who die have significant pulmonary emboli at postmortem examination, and about 15% have massive pulmonary emboli. These emboli are commonly missed, being diagnosed as pneumonia or non-specific deterioration.

Question D   2, 4 and 5 are correct.

Venography is relatively fast, and can outline almost the whole venous system of a limb at one time. It is probably still the reference method of diagnosis, but is expensive in radiologist's time and has some morbidity. Doppler ultrasound is very quick and convenient as a screening test in these circumstances.

IFS is the most sensitive technique, particularly for small calf vein thromboses. However, it cannot be used above the mid thigh, and therefore, severe proximal thrombi can be missed.

IPG is possibly as sensitive as venography for proximal vein thrombosis, but is not as specific. It is not very sensitive for calf vein thrombosis, and is very difficult to use in stroke victims because of reflex movements.

DU is probably the simplest screening test for DVT, and in both of these patients could have been used to exclude (or prove) massive venous occlusion. It is more sensitive than IPG for calf thromboses, but less so than IFS.

For those without access to more specialised investigations, venography remains the investigation of choice.

Question E   3 and 5 are correct.

Subcutaneous heparin is absorbed irregularly in elderly females. Five thousand units 12 hourly would underdose about 40% of subjects and produce measurable changes in coagulation (i.e. overdose in the context of prophylaxis) in 10%. It is not surprising, therefore, that clinical trials have not found subcutaneous heparin to be very effective prophylaxis for DVT in elderly patients with fractured hips.

There is little evidence that ageing per se increases the risk of bleeding when anticoagulants are used correctly. However, the old may have diseases which predispose to bleeding such as gastric erosion, and this should be borne in mind. In contrast to oral anticoagulants, heparin has been shown to be more risky in elderly females.

Cardiac failure is another predisposing factor for DVT and systemic emboli. Prophylaxis should be considered in some patients.

It is not known if anticoagulants are more hazardous after a stroke; however, if anticoagulants are considered, a CT scan can be used to exclude patients with intracranial haemorrhage as the primary pathology.

After hip surgery, few would disagree that a patient proven to have a DVT by some suitable screening procedure should be anti-coagulated in the usual way. A combination of IFS and IPG or DU is a very effective screening method which is sensitive to proximal and distal thromboses. Some may prefer to rely on the tests for proximal thrombosis alone (IPG or DU).

Suggested further reading

Warlow C et al (1976) Deep venous thrombosis of the legs after strokes. Part I - Incidence of predisposing factors; Part II - Natural history. British Medical Journal, 1, 1178-1183

CASE 24

DIURETIC TREATMENT

HISTORY

Mr A, aged 68 years, was admitted to hospital with shortness of breath. He had been a life-long smoker, and a heavy drinker while in the army as a "regular". After his retirement he lived alone and never consulted his doctor. Examination showed a regular pulse of 100/minute, blood pressure 160/95 mmHg, his heart was clinically enlarged, the jugular veins were engorged and there was moderate ankle and sacral oedema. Careful auscultation of the heart revealed a fourth heart sound and a soft systolic murmur at the apex. He was clinically euthyroid, and the optic fundi were normal.

Investigations showed a normal full blood count (including platelets). The ESR was 13 mm/hour. A chest radiograph showed uniform cardiomegaly and evidence of pulmonary venous hypertension. The blood urea was 15 mmol/l, creatinine 1.24 mmol/l, and the electrolytes were normal. Thyroid function tests showed a T4 of 140 nmol/l and the TSH was less than 1 mu/l.

Question A

Which of the following statements are true?

1. Renal function declines with age.

2. The blood urea and creatinine usually rise above the normal range with age.

3. The approximate glomerular filtration rate can be computed from the patient's weight, age and serum creatinine.

4. Congestive cardiac failure is the commonest cause of an elevated blood urea in the elderly.

5. Treatment of heart failure usually improves renal function.

Question B

If allowed to examine Mr A again at this stage, what would you look for, and what further investigations would you ask for?

PROGRESS

He was treated with oral frusemide, which improved his symptoms and signs of cardiac failure. However, he developed acute retention of urine, and had a urinary catheter inserted. Rectal examination was unremarkable, as was an intravenous urogram. The blood urea was now 20 mmol/l and creatinine 0.3 mmol/l. A urologist advised that he be catheterised until his medical condition was stablised, and then the catheter withdrawn. After an initial diuresis (4 kg weight loss) he still had episodes of paroxysmal nocturnal dyspnoea. A week later the urea was 25 mmol/l.

Question C

What would you do now?

ANSWERS

Question A   1, 3 and 4 are correct.

Renal plasma flow and glomerular filtration rate fall linearly with age, the latter at a mean rate of about 1 ml/min/year of life (from maturity). However, protein intake and muscle mass also decline with age, and this tends to mask the reduced clearance of urea and creatinine. Thus, although these both tend to rise with age, they do so much less than the rate of renal function declines (which roughly halves between 20 and 75 years). The blood urea and creatinine may still be "normal" when the glomerular filtration rate is below 40 ml/min. They are therefore of little use to make judgements about renal function. Accurate 24-hour urine collection, and labelled ETA clearance studies are often impractical but a fair estimate of glomerular filtration may be made from the serum creatinine, weight and age, either using a nomogram, or the following formula:

Glomerular filtration rate (ml/min) =

$$\frac{(140 - age)}{serum\ creatinine} \times \frac{weight\ (kg)}{72}$$

Congestive cardiac failure is probably the commonest cause of a mildly elevated blood urea in the elderly but unfortunately treatment with diuretics often reduces the glomerular filtration rate further.

Question B

The two major issues are the cause of the heart failure, and the cause of the elevated urea. With regard to the renal impairment, abdominal palpation to exclude obvious retention is mandatory, as is rectal examination of the prostate. An ultrasound examination of the bladder after micturition (to measure the residual volume) and of the kidneys (to exclude hydronephrosis) is probably the simplest test to exclude an obstructive uropathy. An alternative would be an intravenous urogram.

With regard to the heart failure, valvular heart disease seems unlikely, as does previous hypertension. An ECG may help in further refuting hypertension, and might show evidence of a previous myocardial infarction, or, more likely, non-specific T-wave inversion. T3 toxicosis is still possible, and thiamine deficiency (beri-beri) should be considered in view of the history of heavy drinking.

Question C

The clinical triad of congestive heart failure, a raised blood urea and diuretic treatment is commonly encountered in old age.

It is likely that the diuretic treatment is reducing the cardiac output, and thus affecting renal function. If the patient's heart failure is well controlled it is worth trying to reduce the diuretic dosage, and thus improve renal function. On the other hand, though this man has symptoms due to his heart failure, a further increase in diuretics will aggravate the renal function and probably result in electrolyte disturbances (particularly hyponatraemia).

The addition of a vasodilator, perhaps a nitrate preparation, or an ACE inhibitor (such as captopril or enalapril) should be considered at this stage. Digitalisation could be tried, though the value of this in a patient who is in sinus rhythm is uncertain.

Suggested further reading

Barr M L et al (1977) The effects of discontinuing long-term diuretic therapy in the elderly. Age and Ageing, 6, 38-44

Caird F I, Dall J L C, Kennedy R D (eds.) (1976) Cardiology in Old Age. Plenum Press, New York and London

CASE 25

EPISODES OF UNCONSCIOUSNESS

HISTORY

Mrs L W, aged 74 years, was seen at hospital complaining of black-outs. She had had four in all and though none had been fully witnessed, she had undoubtedly been unconscious. There was no aura, no incontinence, no tongue biting, and she had bruised her-self once. She thought that she remained unconscious for about 10-15 minutes. The four attacks seemed entirely random. Her only medication was temazepam at night. A thorough physical examination was unremarkable. Investigations were reported as follows: ECG - atrial extrasystoles; EEG - diffuse slow wave activity; random blood glucose - 10.6 mmol/l. All the following were normal or negative: full blood count; ESR; WR; chest radiograph; blood urea and electrolytes.

Question A

Which of the following statements are true?

1. Subdural haematomas occasionally present with grand mal epilepsy.

2. Slow wave activity on an EEG is indicative of diffuse cerebral disease.

3. The absence of tongue biting or incontinence makes major epilepsy unlikely in this case.

4. Reactive hypoglycaemia should be excluded.

5. Nocturnal fits sometimes cause early morning confusion.

A glucose tolerance test showed a mildly diabetic pattern with no delayed hypoglycaemia. A therapeutic trial of phenytoin was started but the patient had two further "turns".

Question B

Why might her symptoms have continued?

The serum phenytoin level was satisfactory. A repeat 12-lead ECG was unchanged, but 24-hour ambulant ECG monitoring showed the changes illustrated in Figure 13.

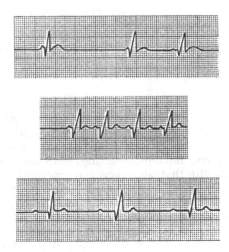

Figure 13 ECG rhythm strips

Question C

What does this ECG show?

Question D

Which of the following statements are true?

1. Ectopic beats (atrial or ventricular) have been detected in up to 40% of routine ECGs in the elderly.

2. Right bundle branch block is more common than left bundle branch block in old age.

3. A reduction in the number of pacemaker cells in the sino-atrial node appears to be a normal ageing phenomenon.

4. A reduction in the cell numbers in the atrioventricular node occurs with ageing.

5. Fibrosis of the bundle of His and the bundle fascicles occurs with ageing.

Question E

Which of the following are true about cardiac rhythm in the elderly?

1. Sinoatrial block may be a prelude to more serious dysrhythmias.

2. 24-hour ECG monitoring shows that cardiac dysrhythmias are as common in the asymptomatic elderly as those with syncope or fainting episodes.

3.   Atrial fibrillation occurs in about 2% of the elderly population.

4.   Supraventricular tachydysrhythmias are more likely to be symptomatic than in the young.

5.   Paroxysmal atrial fibrillation is often not prevented by digoxin.

A permanent pacemaker was inserted and the patient's symptoms disappeared. She was well on follow-up eight years later.

ANSWERS

Question A   1, 4 and 5 are correct.

Subdural haematomas occasionally present with grand mal epilepsy. Slow wave activity on this patient's EEG was likely to be due to the benzodiazepine she had been taking. This effect may take more than a week to disappear after the drug is stopped. The absence of tongue biting and incontinence is of little diagnostic importance. Reactive hypoglycaemia may present with intermittent confusion, unconsciousness or fits. It is more common in the early stages of maturity onset diabetes mellitus, and is thus quite common in the elderly. Nocturnal fits may pass unnoticed, but a history of nocturnal incontinence, or early morning confusion may be helpful.

Question B

In these circumstances, one should consider that the patient may not be taking the medication, that the medication is ineffective or that the diagnosis is wrong (as in this case). Compliance with many drugs can now be checked by measuring drug levels, and this can be very helpful in the management of elderly patients.

Question C

These rhythm strips show episodes of sinoatrial block (no P waves) and episodes of bradycardia and tachycardia. These features are characteristic of the "sick sinus syndrome".

Question D   1, 2, 3 and 5 are correct.

Ectopic beats are very common even in a healthy elderly population; they seem to be of no significance.

In the elderly population as a whole, right bundle branch block is more common than left bundle branch block, though in a hospital population, the incidence of left bundle branch block may be greater because of the presence of disease.

The number of pacemaker cells in the sinoatrial node declines with age, irrespective of the presence of ischaemic heart disease, whereas cells in the atrioventricular node are usually only found to be abnormal in patients with heart disease.

The commonest cause of heart block in the elderly is bilateral bundle branch fibrosis, which seems independent of other cardiac pathology. For this reason, the prognosis of an elderly subject with idiopathic heart block is very good once a pacemaker is inserted.

Question E   All are correct.

Sinoatrial block may indicate the sick sinus syndrome (as in this patient) which is more common in the elderly, probably because of the cellular changes in the SA node.

Several studies have shown that cardiac dysrhythmias correlate poorly with "turns" in patients who have both, and indeed, are nearly as common in asymptomatic subjects as in patients. An example of this would be atrial fibrillation.

Atrial tachycardias are more serious in the elderly than in the young because of reduced cardiac reserve. With fast heart rates, the cardiac output may fall because of poor ventricular filling; this effect is greater in old people. Atrial fibrillation with a ventricular rate of 180/minute can produce syncope in some old people.

Paroxysmal atrial fibrillation commonly is not controlled by digoxin; a variety of alternatives have been suggested, such as verapamil, amiodarone and quinidine.

Suggested further reading

Caird F I, Dall J L C, Kennedy R D (eds.) (1976) Cardiology in Old Age. Plenum Press, New York and London

Caird F I et al (1974) Significance of abnormalities of the electrocardiogram in old people. British Heart Journal, 36, 1912-1918

Campbell A E et al (1974) Prevalence of abnormalities of the electrocardiogram in old people. British Heart Journal, 36, 1005-1011

CASE 26

LOSS OF VISION IN ONE EYE

HISTORY

A 77-year-old lady was seen in the outpatient department complaining of episodes of weakness of the right leg, sometimes accompanied by clumsiness of the right hand. She described three such episodes which had occurred in the preceding month; the symptoms began suddenly and on each occasion had resolved completely within about 30 minutes. She did not notice any visual loss or speech impairment at any time. She did not lose consciousness.

Physical examination, including blood pressure, was normal.

Question A

Which is the most likely diagnosis?

1. Vertebrobasilar insufficiency

2. Transient ischaemic attacks

3. Todd's paresis

4. Non-disabling strokes

5. Spinal cord ischaemia at cervical level

Question B

Are there any investigations which are likely to lead to a firm diagnosis in this patient?

MANAGEMENT

The presumptive diagnosis of left hemispherical transient ischaemic attacks was made and treatment was started with aspirin, 300 mg daily. A full blood count, blood urea, electrolytes and ECG were normal.

Question C

Do you have any criticisms of this treatment?

Question D

Which of the following is true?

1. Anticoagulation is never indicated for transient ischaemic attacks.

2. Carotid endarterectomy has been shown to greatly reduce the risk of a completed stroke in patients having hemispherical transient ischaemic attacks.

3. Aspirin should be the treatment of choice only in those patients not suitable for carotid endarterectomy.

4. Completed stroke is a complication of carotid endarterectomy.

5. Aspirin should not be given for the treatment of transient ischaemic attacks in people over 75 years of age.

A YEAR LATER

The patient was admitted urgently with a history of sudden loss of vision in the left eye the previous day, without improvement between onset and admission. She had a mild occipital headache, present since the loss of vision, but no history of preceding headache or amaurosis fugax. She had remained on aspirin and had only experienced about four episodes of transient right-sided weakness over the past year, the last one several weeks before the loss of vision.

ON EXAMINATION

The heart, chest, abdomen and CNS were normal. Vision in the right eye was normal, and completely lost in the left eye. The pupils reacted bilaterally when light was shone in the right eye, but not at all when shone in the left. The right optic fundus was normal. The left was generally pale with some patches of congestion and few vessels could be seen; the left optic disc had a less distinct margin than the right.

Question E

The lesion is likely to be in:

1. the visual cortex

2. the left optic radiation

3. the right internal capsule

4. the left optic nerve or retina

5. a partial lesion of the optic chiasma

Question F

What are the most important diagnoses to consider?

How would you support or prove the diagnosis?

Question G

What is the treatment and how does it influence the prognosis for vision?

Question H   Which are true?

Giant cell arteritis:

1. is commoner in white people than in black people.

2. can always be diagnosed with certainty by muscle biopsy.

3. frequently causes raised serum muscle enzymes when polymyalgia rheumatica is present.

4. can only be diagnosed with certainty by arterial biopsy.

5. can cause a hypoproliferative anaemia which resolves when corticosteroid treatment is given.

Question I   Which are true?

Giant cell arteritis:

1. is much commoner in women.

2. should be considered in a patient with pyrexia of unknown origin.

3. is associated with a normal electromyelogram when polymyalgia rheumatica is present.

4. invariably requires lifelong maintenance corticosteroid treatment.

5. The marked rise in ESR is caused by raised blood gamma-globulin and fibrinogen levels.

ANSWERS

Question A   2

The symptoms suggest episodes of left cerebral hemisphere dysfunction. When these are of less than 24 hours duration, they are likely to be caused by temporary complete or partial arterial occlusion by platelet emboli and are called transient ischaemic attacks. When such episodes persist for more than 24 hours they are usually referred to as minor strokes.

Vertebrobasilar insufficiency and high cervical cord ischaemia would both usually give rise to bilateral symptoms, though unilateral symptoms and signs can occur.

Todd's paresis is the temporary hemiparesis or monoparesis which can follow a convulsion; there is almost always a history of a grand mal or Jacksonian seizure. The paresis usually persists for longer than 30 minutes and is often accompanied by other post-ictal

139

features such as perplexity, confusion and temporary extensor plantar responses.

Question B

No, the diagnosis relies on the history. Angiography may show carotid arterial disease, such as atheromatous stenosis, but this does not prove the diagnosis of transient ischaemic attacks. Furthermore, the absence of arteriographic abnormality in the carotid arteries does not refute the diagnosis. Cerebral arteriography and CT head scanning will not provide information which is likely to influence the diagnosis. Cardiac investigations, to detect possible sources of microemboli from the left chambers or valves should be considered in patients with atrial fibrillation, valve lesions, recent myocardial infarction or chronic left ventricular enlargement; echocardiography is non-invasive and provides a reasonable view of the structures concerned. This is not indicated in the patient described, who has no abnormal signs in the cardiovascular system. Before treatment is started the physician should rule out a number of other conditions which may cause or closely mimic transient ischaemic attacks, particularly polycythaemia, anaemia, hypoglycaemia or intracardiac sources of emboli.

Question C

The ideal treatment for transient ischaemic attacks is unknown. It would be reasonable in this case to prescribe aspirin and observe the response; however, theory suggests that a dose as little as 75 mg daily, or even on alternate days, is sufficient to reduce platelet adhesiveness. The dose of 300 mg daily is probably too high, and carries a greater risk of causing gastric bleeding than the smaller dose. However, most trials of aspirin have been at doses of 300 mg daily or more; a trial of low dose aspirin for transient ischaemic attacks is long overdue. It could be argued that such a patient should have carotid angiography, and, if a reasonably localised stenosis is found, a carotid endarterectomy plus aspirin. The evidence in favour of these two approaches is not entirely clear, though extensive trials currently being performed might clarify the matter in the future. There is little evidence in favour of treatment with dipyridamole for transient ischaemic attacks.

Question D   4

Carotid endarterectomy carries a small risk of intra-operative stroke; this is less than 5% in good centres. Furthermore, while some trials have shown a reduction in transient ischaemic attacks and completed strokes after carotid endarterectomy, this improvement is not dramatic, though individuals sometimes benefit considerably. However, it is not true to say that the operation greatly reduces the risk of a completed stroke.

Some authorities consider that aspirin alone should be the treatment only when patients with platelet emboli are not suitable for carotid surgery. Others dispute this, and the results of current trials are awaited.

Low doses of aspirin carry only a very small risk of upper gastrointestinal bleeding and can be given to very aged patients with relative safety. Aspirin at any dose should be used with great caution in patients with a history of peptic ulceration.

Question E 4

The appearance of the optic fundus on the left suggests retinal artery occlusion; this is in keeping with the pattern of the pupillary light reflex abnormality and the complete loss of vision in the left eye.

Visual cortex lesions cause "cortical" blindness which, if unilateral, has some of the features of a homonymous hemianopia but is often denied by the patient.

A left optic radiation lesion causes a right homonymous hemianopia (partial or complete), or quadrantanopia. A right internal capsule lesion causes a left homonymous hemianopia. Optic chiasma lesions cause variable patterns of visual loss, but this cannot explain the entire clinical picture in this patient.

Question F

The most important diagnoses to consider in this context are retinal artery occlusion by platelet embolisation, though this usually causes amaurosis fugax rather than irreversible loss of vision, and giant cell arteritis, which should always be included in the differential diagnosis of sudden monocular blindness in elderly people. Other causes of monocular blindness are much less likely in this case, in view of the appearance of the retina.

An ESR should be performed immediately. If it is high, the diagnosis of giant cell arteritis should be considered the most likely until proved otherwise. A temporal artery biopsy can make the diagnosis definite, if inflammatory infiltration and giant cells are seen.

Question G

Corticosteroid treatment causes a dramatic improvement in the arteritis; prednisolone in initial doses of 40-60 mg daily should be given, then reduced progressivly as symptoms and the ESR are monitored. Unfortunately, useful improvement in vision rarely occurs. Some physicians advocate the use of intravenous dextran in the acute stage of blindness due to cranial arteritis; this is said to re-establish retinal perfusion in some cases, though the value of this treatment is not certain. Platelet aggregation in the inflamed arteries may be an important part of the pathological process leading to retinal artery occlusion, so a case can be made for giving low

141

dose aspirin in the acute phase; it is noteworthy that some clinicians have reported an excess of transient ischaemic attacks in patients with giant cell arteritis. The pain of temporal arteritis usually responds to paracetamol, though analgesic doses of aspirin can be used considering the arguments outlined above.

Question H   1, 4 and 5 are true.

Studies of giant cell arteritis in the USA indicate that whites have a much higher incidence of the condition compared with blacks.

Muscle biopsy specimens can contain small arteries which have the characteristic changes of giant cell arteritis; this method is un-reliable and has a high false negative rate.

In contrast to polymyositis, polymyalgia rheumatica does not cause a rise in serum muscle enzymes.

Arterial biopsy in this condition can be diagnostic when giant cells are seen in an inflamed vessel wall; corticosteroid treatment can reverse these changes within days. No other test gives a firm diagnostic result.

A normochromic normocytic anaemia occurs in giant cell arter-itis, particularly if the onset has been relatively insidious. There is a rapid improvement when steroid treatment is given, and a persist-ing anaemia should prompt a search for another cause.

Question I   2, 3 and 5 are true.

The incidence is probably almost equal in both sexes, though some authors state a moderately higher incidence in women.

Pyrexia is not a common feature of giant cell arteritis, but is occasionally the presenting abnormality, hence giant cell arteritis should be considered in an elderly patient with a PUO.

The electromyogram is normal in polymyalgia rheumatica.

The length of time for which steroid should be given in this condition is not known, and there is no doubt that patients vary considerably in this respect. Some do require a lifelong maintenance dose to prevent relapse, though many can be weaned off steroid within 2 years of the diagnosis.

A high ESR is usually caused by an increase in the ratio of heavy proteins to albumin; in giant cell arteritis the gamma-globulins and fibrinogen are raised.

Suggested further reading

Hander G C, Allen G L (1978-79) Giant cell arteritis: a review. Bulletin of Rheumatic Diseases, 29, 980-986

Isaacs B (1985) The central nervous system - stroke. In: Brocklehurst J C (ed.) Textbook of Geriatric Medicine and Gerontology, 3rd Edn. Churchill Livingstone, Edin-burgh

Millikan C (1979) The transient ischaemic attack. Advances in Neurology, 25, 135-140

Parkin P J et al (1982) Amaurosis fugax: some aspects of management. Journal of Neurology, Neurosurgery and Psychiatry, 45, 1-6

CASE 27

TEAMWORK

The physician in geriatric medicine cannot work alone. For a department to function to the patient's best advantage, it is essential to harness the expertise of a number of individuals, and coordinate their efforts. The physician needs to have a reasonable working knowledge of the content of these individual's work so as to maintain a birdseye view of the department as a whole; this chapter will test your grasp of this.

Question A

List the types of staff you consider to be essential for the effective running of a geriatric rehabilitation ward. Outline briefly the content of their work.

Question B

List the types of staff you consider to be desirable, but not essential, as part-time or visiting members of your rehabilitation team.

Question C

It is reasonable to staff geriatric rehabilitation wards with nurses who are largely untrained (auxillary nurses), under the supervision of a ward sister. Discuss.

Question D

Which of the following can be part of the occupational therapist's work on the geriatric rehabilitation ward?

1. Performing tests for dyspraxia

2. Teaching hemiplegics to transfer from chair to toilet

3. Pre-discharge home visits with the patient

4. Reducing dependence on mechanical aids to a minimum

5. Observing the patient for signs of depression

Question E

The Activities of Daily Living (ADL) are considered to be essential for patients to lead a relatively independent life; what are they?

143

Example

A 68-year-old right hemiparetic man has been in the geriatric rehabilitation ward for 3 weeks. His power loss is minimal and his physiotherapy has progressed to the point where he can walk un-aided except for a pole in his right hand. He finds it difficult to communicate because of his aphasia. However, he lives alone and the problems which are delaying his discharge are his inability to dress himself and a tendency for food to fall from his mouth while he is chewing.

Question F

Despite a good return of power in the right limbs, he is unable to dress himself; what is the most likely reason for this? How might this be assessed?

Question G

Which member of your team should be asked to help him with his chewing and drooling?

Question H

Speech therapists are of no proven value in stroke rehabilitation. Discuss.

Question I

With which other member(s) of the team is each of the named therapists below likely to work most closely in the following sets of circumstances?

1. The physiotherapist dealing with a semiconscious patient 48 hours after a severe left hemiplegia.

2. The physiotherapist dealing with an elderly immobile patient who has had several strokes affecting both sides, and who is awaiting placement in a continuing care bed.

3. The physiotherapist who is making no headway with a patient with Parkinson's disease with severe bradykinesia.

4. The occupational therapist who is concerned about a patient's performance in the kitchen.

5. The occupational therapist whose work with a particular patient has to be constantly interrupted because the patient is often incontinent of faeces.

6. The speech therapist who is trying to teach an aphasic right hemiplegic to use a signboard for basic communication.

7. The medical social worker who is uncertain about which modifications will be needed in the house of an amputee before discharge from hospital.

8. The physiotherapist who cannot pinpoint the reason for lack of progress in a hemiplegic with relatively little power loss, sensory or perceptual impairment.

9. The staff nurse caring for hemiplegic patients for the first time on a rehabilitation ward, who is uncertain how to assist patients in transferring from bed to chair.

10. The ward sister who notices that a patient takes a long time to swallow a mouthful of food, and tends to cough when drinking warm fluids.

ANSWERS

Question A

In addition to junior medical staff, a consultant geriatrician will require the following staff to run a rehabilitation ward effectively.

1. Nurses. Ideally, the nurse in charge will have a special interest in rehabilitation, and should be encouraged to attend courses on the care of the elderly. The nursing staff have greater continuity in their contact with the patients than any of the other members of the rehabilitation team; they are in a key position to relay problems which arise to the geriatrician. As well as carrying out the usual nursing work on the ward, the nurses will need to liaise closely with the other therapists so that certain aspects of physiotherapy and occupational therapy can be performed by the nurses out of normal working hours and at weekends, thus avoiding gaps in treatment. The ward nursing staff also liaise with the district nurses who might need to visit patients after discharge. The broad nature of nursing on a rehabilitation ward makes it a suitable environment for student nurses.

2. Physiotherapist. A physiotherapist is needed with a good background of general physiotherapy and preferably, experience in geriatric rehabilitation or on a stroke unit. The physiotherapist will assess a patient's locomotor disorder, plan a reasonable sequence of physiotherapy, and liaise closely with the geriatrician and other staff.

3. Occupational therapist. While occupational therapists can be said to be non-essential staff on general medical wards, this is not the case on rehabilitation wards where they are vital. The occupational therapist needs to be able to devote her time to the rehabilitation ward in order to be effective, and will work closely with the physiotherapist throughout the period of in-patient rehabilitation. The occupational therapist will also advise on the need for various aids and devices, and will

often be involved in deciding which, if any, modifications to the patient's home might be needed before discharge from hospital.

4. Medical social worker. A large proportion of elderly patients need help from the medical social worker at the time they are in-patients. A medical social worker with particular experience with the elderly is ideal. The medical social worker can give help with benefits, allowances, pensions, housing and legal matters, and will often be asked by patients or their families to assist in arranging placement in a rest home, nursing home or local authority elderly persons home. The medical social worker frequently works closely with the occupational therapist when arrangements have to be made to modify a patient's home. The medical social worker liaises between the rehabilitation team and the local social services department to organise home-helps, meals-on-wheels, laundry service, community wardens, day centres, luncheon clubs and so on, as well as the various voluntary services, such as stroke clubs.

5. Speech therapist. The authors consider the speech therapist to be an essential part of a complete geriatric rehabilitation team, though some authorities might disagree. The speech therapist is of special importance when patients have had strokes. They delineate the nature of the patient's speech problems and treat accordingly, often employing alternative means of communication such as picture charts and sign language. The speech therapist can often be of great help when the patient has difficulty with swallowing or a tendency to dribble.

Question B

1. Dietitian. Reducing diets are occasionally needed, though they are seldom really effective in the obese elderly patient with poor mobility. Dietary advice for patients with diabetes, renal failure and habitual constipation makes up most of the remainder. The speech therapist and dietitian sometimes need to work together on a suitable diet for stroke patients with swallowing problems.

2. Chiropodist. A considerable amount of morbidity in the elderly population is related to minor foot disorders; patients can, for instance, have their mobility severely restricted by a painful callous. Many of these problems can be rectified by chiropody. The need is even greater in the elderly diabetic who is particularly at risk from foot infections, digital gangrene, and sensory neuropathy leading to unnoticed foot trauma.

Question C

In the early days of geriatric medicine many wards were staffed by relatively untrained nurses; this was not satisfactory, and there can be little doubt that the standard of nursing care, as well as the general ambience of the wards, has improved since the proportion of trained staff has risen. The English National Board organises various courses which staff can attend to improve their knowledge of the problems of the elderly. Happily, many young nurses now see geriatric departments, particularly rehabilitation wards, as a challenging environment in which to develop their careers.

Question D   1, 2, 3, 4 and 5

The occupational therapist will perform tests to detect and illustrate dyspraxia in hemiplegics; with particular emphasis on dyspraxias which interfere with the practical aspects of the patient's rehabilitation. This information is often useful to the physiotherapist who may find that limb dyspraxia is hindering locomotor rehabilitation.

Transferring between bed, chair and toilet is central to a patient's independence. The teaching of transfers is often regarded as the province of the physiotherapist, though occupational therapists often need to take an active part in this aspect of rehabilitation, particularly when modifications to the patient's bed, chair or toilet might be necessary.

A visit to the patient's home by the occupational therapist before discharge will often be required in order to predict the level of independence which the patient will need to attain before discharge, and to organise any aids or modifications in advance. Usually, this home visit is done with the patient so that a realistic assessment of the patient's disabilities and requirements can be made in situ. The occupational therapist and medical social worker will liaise with the social services rehabilitation officer when structural alterations or equipment are required for the patient's home.

A huge array of mechanical aids, simple and complex, are available. Used properly, they can be of immense help to the disabled elderly. However, aids can be misplaced, lost or broken, and the more complicated ones can malfunction; most can be seen as badges of disability. Therefore, the physiotherapist and occupational therapist will try to minimise a patient's dependence on mechanical aids by imaginative therapy aimed at helping the patient to cope by utilising residual function, and thoughtful adjustments to lifestyle and environment.

All the staff on the rehabilitation team should be looking out for signs of depression, which can markedly hamper the patient's progress if it is neglected. For instance, tearfulness during a dressing practice session could be the earlist sign of a rising sense of helplessness in a hemiplegic.

Question E

The Activities of Daily Living (ADL) in the context of geriatric rehabilitation are:

1.   Mobility - to live alone a patient really needs to be able to transfer between bed, chair and commode without help

2.   Dressing

3.   Toilet

4.   Feeding

These are the bare necessities; the amount of outside help a patient will need will depend on how far the definition of these activities extends. For instance, to live alone a person really needs to be able to prepare basic food and drinks, but if other people bring all the meals in, this will not be necessary.

Question F

He is probably either dyspraxic, that is, unable to perform the necessary integrated sequence of movements required to perform a relatively complex task such as putting on clothes, or has central sensory neglect of the right side of the body with the result that he cannot appreciate and utilise spatial relationships on that side. Both of these can seriously hamper dressing, and both will tend to be made worse by a hemianopia or by a receptive aphasia which prevents the patient understanding the commands of the therapists. If there is any doubt the geriatrician should repeat the neurological examination to look for evidence of sensory neglect, and arrange for the occupational therapist to perform formal tests for dyspraxia.

Question G

The speech therapist usually incorporates the treatment of chewing and swallowing problems into her regimen for the hemiplegic patient. The improvement in lip seal required for the hemiplegic to enunciate some consonants also reduces the tendency to drool. The nurses are often the first to notice the less obvious examples of this. Physiotherapists also have treatment routines for patients with facial palsy.

Question H

Some studies have shown that the speech of aphasic hemiplegics, when assessed a year after the stroke, is not influenced by speech therapy given during the recovery phase; this is sometimes used in arguments against the use of speech therapists in geriatric rehabilitation. However, this presupposes that speech therapists only try to teach aphasics to speak again, which is far from the real pattern of their work. For instance, the speech therapist can often improve overall communication with a dysphasic patient by means of picture charts, sign language and facial expression. As already mentioned, they provide valuable treatment for patients with swallowing, drooling and chewing difficulties. They are often the first members of the team to detect the subtler levels of a confusional state, a mood disorder, an early dementia or minor degrees of dyspraxia. They also work with patients other than hemiplegics; for example, patients with dysphonia due to Parkinson's disease.

Question I

1. The physiotherapist will work closely with the nursing staff when a patient with a recent hemiplegia is still semi-conscious, in order to start positioning the limbs properly from this early stage. This approach is thought to lead to better control of spasticity and a lower incidence of shoulder subluxation later. The nurses will be taking particular care to avoid pressure necrosis at this time.

2. Again, the physiotherapist will need to work with the nurses looking after the multiple bilateral hemiplegic. In such a patient, the physiotherapist will advise on positioning, and perhaps passive exercises to reduce spasticity and hence deformity and pain. The patient will probably be very immobile and the nurses can often glean useful advice from the physiotherapist as to how to best handle the patient during transfers or bathing, for instance.

3. In this case, the physiotherapist should draw the geriatrician's attention to the patient's bradykinesia; a change in drug therapy might be needed.

4. The occupational therapist would need to approach various members of the team in such a case, depending on why the patient could not cope in the kitchen. For instance, if the patient becomes dizzy when standing, the geriatrician should be informed. If the patient is tripping, the physiotherapist would need to consider what might be done to improve matters. If persistent inability to manage in the kitchen is likely to prevent the patient returning home, then the whole team will need to discuss the need for, perhaps, alternative accommodation.

5. The faecal incontinence should be investigated by the geriatrician and treated accordingly. If, for example, a patient with multi-infarct dementia is passing formed stools into the clothes each morning, an arrangement can be made between the occupational therapist and the nurses to give the patient a suppository and empty the bowel before dressing practice is attempted. The patient's attendants might need to continue this treatment after discharge.

6. The patient will use a signboard to communicate with the nurses more than any other member of the team, so the speech therapist should involve the nurses at an early stage. The patient's relatives should also be given an opportunity to learn how best to use a signboard.

7. The medical social worker, occupational therapist and patient should visit the house together and decide what alterations, if any, are needed.

8. The hemiplegic who is not doing well, for no obvious reason, is a fairly frequent problem in a rehabilitation ward. The physiotherapist is often the team member who notices the poor progress first, probably because she stresses the patient physically more than the other team members. The physiotherapist should bring the problem to the attention of the geriatrician. Intercurrent illnesses, such as chest or urinary infections, anaemia, pain or poorly controlled diabetes need to be sought and dealt with. The patient might be depressed, or might have domestic worries which the medical social worker can look into.

9. The physiotherapist on a rehabilitation ward should always be prepared to teach new staff how to handle hemiplegic patients. Proper handling by the nurses will help avoid slips and falls, and painful subluxed shoulders. Patients feel more secure and therefore do better if they are handled properly.

10. The sister should inform the geriatrician and the speech therapist, who between them will decide the reason for the patient's swallowing problem and plan appropriate treatment.

Suggested further reading

Andrews K (1985) Rehabilitation. In: Brocklehurst J C (ed.) Textbook of Geriatric Medicine and Gerontology, 3rd Edn. Churchill Livingstone, Edinburgh

CASE 28

FAECAL INCONTINENCE

HISTORY

A dirty and dishevelled woman of 79 presented to the out-patient department with a history of faecal soiling for a number of weeks which her general practitioner thought was due to severe haemorrhoids. It was difficult to get a very coherent history. She lived alone and had obviously been neglecting herself for some time. She herself denied faecal incontinence but said that she tended to be constipated, although further questioning suggested that this was intermittent rather than a continuing problem. She took Dorbanex from time to time. The haemorrhoids were painful and she generally noticed some blood in the stool. She said she had a good appetite and was provided with meals-on-wheels four times a week, but further questioning suggested that she often left a good deal of these.

She had never married and had worked as a cleaner until she was in her middle 60s. She seemed to be an isolated individual who saw little of her neighbours.

On examination her hair was dark and unkempt, her face pale and slightly puffy with a good deal of facial hair. She showed some **erythema ab igne** on the front of her legs and on the back of her hands and there was minimal pitting oedema. The pulse was 68/minute and regular. Blood pressure 120/70 mmHg. There was no abnormality in the respiratory system. The patient's underclothes showed marked faecal staining. On abdominal examination there were some firm masses palpable in the left iliac fossa and the caecum was soft and palpable. No other abnormalities were identified.

Question A

Discuss:

1. The differential diagnosis.

2. What further investigations should be carried out or ordered in the outpatient department?

3. What are the possible causes of faecal incontinence in this case?

INVESTIGATIONS

Rectal examination

There were florid prolapsing haemorrhoids with a granular appearance. The rectum contained a large quantity of soft faeces and above the rectum some harder masses were palpable which seemed to

151

be indentable. A polyp on a short stalk was palpable just above the anal margin.

Haematology

Haemoglobin 9.5 g/dl, MCV 87 fl, MCH 29.4 pg

Thyroid function tests

T3   0.9 nmol/l

T4   Total - 45 nmol/l   Free - 8 pmol/l

TSH   4 mU/l

Question B

In view of the investigations reported above, which of the following statements are true?

1.   A firm diagnosis of hypothyroidism can be made.

2.   A TRH stimulation test should be carried out.

3.   Treatment should be started with thyroxine at a dose of 0.1 mg per day.

4.   The haematology findings are not consistent with iron deficiency anaemia in this case.

5.   The haematology findings are not consistent with anaemia due to hypothyroidism in this case.

Question C

This patient has an adenomatous polyp of the rectum (tubular adenoma). In this disease which of the following statements are true?

1.   It is a benign lesion and should be removed only if it is causing symptoms.

2.   Biopsy is essential.

3.   It commonly co-exists with colorectal cancer in the elderly.

4.   Colonoscopy or barium enema is mandatory.

5.   Malignancy rate for adenomatous polyp is about 5%.

ANSWERS

Question A

1.   The differential diagnoses in this patient include:

Hypothyroidism - from the appearance of general neglect, the puffiness of the face, **erythema ab igne**, increase in facial hair. The pulse of 68/minute and blood pressure of 120/70 mmHg are consistent with such a diagnosis although they might also both be lower.

Organic disease of the colon or rectum, particularly carcinoma - in view of the presenting symptom of faecal incontinence and the apparent history of constipation.

Depression - this is suggested by the same features as those of hypothyroidism with which it may be associated. Constipation is also a somatic feature of depression. The patient's rather isolated lifestyle and past history are additional features supporting such a diagnosis.

Dementia - this may be suggested by the patient's appearance of neglect, the patchy history which is available and the denial of faecal incontinence. Chronic brain failure is occasionally caused by hypothyroidism. More commonly, senile dementia of Alzheimer's type and hypothyroidism may co-exist.

Haemorrhoids - from the history.

Anaemia - from the general appearance and the fact that haemorrhoids predispose to iron deficiency anaemia, and hypothyroidism to a macrocytic anaemia.

2. Investigations

Rectal examination is essential and proctoscopy may also be carried out in the outpatient department. These may indicate the need for subsequent colonoscopy or barium enema. In this patient's case, in order to obtain proper preparation for these, admission to hospital overnight at least would be desirable.

Thyroid function tests.

Full blood count.

Further history is necessary to discover what the patient's mental state has been like over the past few months and years and this should be sought from a relative if one can be located or from the Social Services Department who are likely to be involved since she is receiving meals-on-wheels.

A Social Report is necessary both towards obtaining a full history and also to deal with the dirty and neglected house which is almost certainly associated with the patient's state.

3. Incontinence of faeces in old people has three major causes:

(a) Constipation leading to retention of faeces with overflow incontinence (the terminal reservoir syndrome).

(b) Organic disease of the rectum and colon particularly if this causes episodes of diarrhoea or impairs the closing mechanisms at the anorectal area.

153

(c)   Chronic brain failure due, for instance, to space-occupying lesion, dementia or normal pressure hydrocephalus and which impairs the patient's ability to inhibit reflex defaecation taking place after a mass peristaltic movement.

In the present case there is reason to suspect:

(a)   Constipation because of the clinical findings: the possible diagnosis of hypothyroidism or depression; the rather vague history of constipation and the fact that the patient takes a laxative.

(b)   An organic disease in the colon or rectum cannot be excluded at this stage and requires further investigation. The laxative itself may cause diarrhoea and precipitate faecal incontinence. Haemorrhoids do not usually of themselves produce faecal incontinence but if painful, may lead to chronic constipation and overflow incontinence. This is also possible in view of the possible diagnosis of chronic brain failure.

Question B 1 is correct.

A firm diagnosis of hypothyroidism can be made in the presence of a low total T4 level, particularly in association with a history consistent with this disease. The fact that the T3 level is within normal limits does not rule out hypothyroidism since there is some overlap with normal and there may be a compensatory increase of T3. However, in the presence of low T4 and an elevated TSH a clear diagnosis can be made.

Elevated TSH values without low serum T4 may occur in old age and should this be the case, some further investigation is required which may include a TRH test or serum assay for thyroid antibodies.

A dose of thyroxine of 0.1 mg is satisfactory for maintenance levels but in old people the drug must be introduced gradually and a dose of 0.025 mg in the first place is appropriate. As far as the anaemia is concerned, it may be suspected clinically that this patient would have both loss of iron (from bleeding from the haemorrhoids) and the anaemia of hypothyroidism which is usually macrocytic due to the absence of thyroxine as a contributory factor in haematopoiesis. These therefore tend to produce opposite effects on red cells (microcytosis in iron deficiency and macrocytosis in hypothyroidism) and a normocytic normochromic picture in the presence of both of these diseases is not inconsistent with either.

Question C 1, 3, 4 and 5 are correct.

An adenomatous polyp of itself is benign but is potentially malignant (with a malignancy rate of about 5%). For this reason it must be removed both to establish whether or not it is actually malignant and also because of its possibility of showing malignant changes later. Adenomas in the rectum have been noted in 95% of rectums removed for carcinoma and 20% of all patients with carcinoma have other tumours (malignant or benign) in the lower bowel. An adenomatous polyp commonly co-exists with colorectal cancer and colonoscopy or barium meal is mandatory.

In this case, as is so often so with old people, the faecal incontinence may have had more than one cause. The patient's hypothyroidism was treated and as a result of this, she became much more clear mentally and after her house had been restored by the Home-help Department she was able to maintain it in good order. Her constipation cleared up. She also had the adenomatous polyp removed and it was benign on biopsy. The haemorrhoids were treated by injection with a reasonable result. It is likely that the constipation and the polyp just above the anal margin were both contributing to her faecal incontinence and this also was no longer a problem after her treatment was complete. Sigmoidoscopy and barium enema showed no evidence of malignancy or other adenomas in the colon but she should be kept under surveillance and faecal occult blood tests carried out every year with further investigation should they prove positive.

Suggested further reading

Brocklehurst J C (1985) Colonic disease in the elderly. In: James D (ed.) Clinics in Gastroenterology Vol.14/no.4. Gastrointestinal Disorders in the Elderly. W.B. Saunders Co. Ltd., London

CASE 29

DOUBLE INCONTINENCE

HISTORY

An 85-year-old woman has been a patient in a long-stay geriatric ward for the last year because of her physical disability associated with bilateral strokes. Over the whole of this time, she has had frequent episodes of faecal incontinence which have been very resistant to a series of attempts at treatment. She also has urinary incontinence which is reasonably managed by regular toiletting.

Her admission to hospital on this occasion was precipitated by a left hemiparesis. She had had a right hemiparesis 1 year earlier but after a relatively short hospital admission with rehabilitation in the geriatric unit, had been able to return home where she lived on her own, being independent in mobility, but very slow. She had urgency of micturition after this first admission and on one occasion was treated for a urinary tract infection with some improvement in the urgency, but it remained a problem and she had occasional episodes of wetting. Her toilet had been specially adapted to cope with the disability of her right side and she found that Kanga pants were helpful to her although she had tried Maxi pads with elastic stretch knickers and found these unsatisfactory. She had occasional episodes of diarrhoea during this time at home and, in fact, had tended to have these on and off for 2 or 3 years. Only occasionally, however, did they cause faecal incontinence if she was unable to get to the toilet in time.

After the second stroke and the left hemiparesis she had total and uncontrolled incontinence of both urine and faeces during her first 3 weeks in hospital. Both of these had improved after rehabilitation. The urinary incontinence had been investigated by urodynamic assessment during her period of rehabilitation and before she became a long-stay patient. The faecal incontinence had been investigated by sigmoidoscopy and barium enema but the only abnormality seen was moderate diverticulosis of the sigmoid colon. The faecal incontinence become progressively worse during her time in the long-stay ward. She passed many frequent, small, loose stools and without treatment she tended to have diarrhoea. During the past year she had had mid-stream specimens of urine examined on four occasions and each showed significant bacteriuria with more than ten white cells. The organism on each occasion was E.coli.

She remained mentally clear but unable to walk. She was able to propel herself in a wheelchair with some difficulty. She needed the assistance of two nurses to get out of bed.

Her previous history had included a diagnosis of angina with occasional treatment by glyceryl trinitrate. A gall stone had been removed 10 years previously and carcinoma of the cervix treated with radiotherapy 5 years previously.

Question A

1. What is the differential diagnosis in this case of the cause of urinary incontinence?

2. What is the differential diagnosis in this case of the cause of faecal incontinence?

Question B

What changes might the occupational therapist have made in the patient's home?

Question C

True or false?

Urodynamic assessment:

1. should be carried out in all elderly patients presenting with incontinence.

2. may sometimes cause bacteraemia.

3. should be carried out in all cases with urge incontinence.

4. should be carried out in all cases of stress incontinence before surgical treatment of the latter is contemplated.

5. is never helpful in 80-year-olds.

Question D

Urinary tract infection:

1. may cause urge incontinence.

2. should always be treated even in long-stay patients whose only symptom is urinary incontinence.

3. reinfection rather than relapse is more likely in this case.

4. continuous prophylaxis with low dose trimethoprim might well be useful in this case.

5. is found in about 20% of institutionalised old people.

Question E

Might any of the following drugs be seriously considered for therapeutic trial in this patient? Write a brief note on each.

1. imipramine
2. metronidazole
3. methyl cellulose
4. codeine phosphate
5. phenoxylate hydrochloride

157

Question F

What would be the advantages or disadvantages of each of the following appliances (a) for this patient and (b) in the general management of urinary incontinence?

1.   Kylie sheet

2.   Maxi-plus pad with stretch knickers

3.   Kanga pants

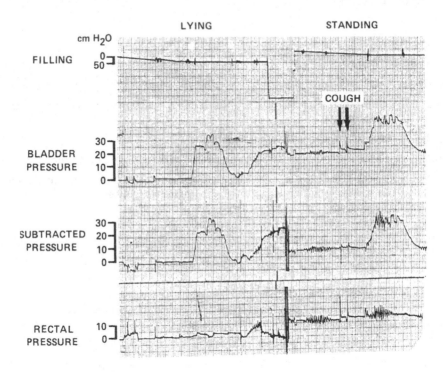

Figure 14 Cystometrogram

Question G

The diagnosis to be made from the cystometrogram shown in Figure 14 is:

1.   detrusor instability

2.   an atonic neurogenic bladder

3.   an uninhibited neurogenic bladder

4.   contracted bladder due to radiotherapy

5.   autonomous neurogenic bladder

ANSWERS

Question A

1. The onset of urinary incontinence at the time of the right hemiparesis and its continuation since then suggests that the precipitating factor was her stroke. This may have been causative in one of two different ways:

    (a) The infarct may have involved the cortical bladder centre in the cyngulate gyrus or its connections and have caused an uninhibited neurogenic bladder.

    (b) Incontinence may have been due to impairment of consciousness and her enforced immobility at the time of the stroke and have continued because of her slowness in walking and getting to the toilet.

    In either of these cases she may well have been predisposed to incontinence by the effects of normal ageing on the cerebral cortex diminishing the effectiveness of cortical inhibition and allowing the sacral bladder reflex arc to escape from higher control, so producing an uninhibited neurogenic bladder.

    While these are by far the most likely causes in view of the history, there may be other contributory causes including the presence of urinary tract infection and the effect of radiation on the bladder itself. Acute cystitis may trigger off incontinence in a bladder which already has impaired inhibition but it is more likely that the recurrent infections recorded in this patient would be incidental, probably caused by the faecal soiling and possibly contributed to by a degree of residual urine. The presence of an uninhibited neurogenic bladder would be demonstrated on urodynamic assessment by cystometry. The effect of radiation could be to further diminish the bladder capacity and perhaps impair complete emptying allowing a significant quantity of residual urine to accumulate.

2. Faecal incontinence may be secondary to constipation due to her immobility and the diarrhoea could be paradoxical diarrhoea associated with faecal impaction. This diagnosis, however, would probably have been made on sigmoidoscopy and barium enema and the incontinence successfully treated thereafter. It is most probable therefore, that the effect of radiation has been to produce the continual diarrhoea and that this is the cause of her faecal incontinence.

Question B

The occupational therapist would have assessed the patient's mobility and environment. In the toilet she may have provided grab handles or a pole accessible to the patient's left hand, a frame around the toilet by which she may have supported herself with both hands and a raised toilet seat to make it easier to get on and off. The toilet paper holder should have been transferred to the left side. Since the patient's mobility was slow, the occupational therapist may have suggested a commode or chemical toilet to be in the bedroom in addition to the changes made in the toilet.

Question C   2 and 4 are correct.

It is impracticable to carry out urodynamic assessment on all old people since those with moderate and severe dementia will almost certainly not co-operate sufficiently for a valid test to be performed. Also, since 80% of urge incontinence is caused by an unstable, uninhibited neurogenic bladder, it is very often appropriate to carry out a trial of therapy with timed voiding and anticholinergic drugs before proceeding to urodynamic assessment in these cases. Similarly, urodynamic assessment may not be needed in patients with retention due to constipation or bladder outlet obstruction or due to the side-effect of drugs. Patients with acute cystitis or senile vaginitis should be treated for these conditions before any urodynamic assessment is carried out. Patients with red cells only in their urine should be cystoscoped at once.

Urodynamic assessment may cause bacteraemia in the elderly and should be covered by an antibiotic "umbrella". This is particularly important in the presence of cardiac valvular lesions. Stress incontinence may be due to pelvic floor weakness and require surgery if it cannot be treated by pelvic floor exercises. However, patients with unstable bladders (detrusor instability) may also present as stress incontinence because the sudden rise of intra-abdominal pressure on coughing or moving sets off a bladder contraction. In such cases, surgical treatment will probably be inappropriate and for this reason, should always be preceded by urodynamic assessment.

Age over 80 is no bar to the appropriate treatment of incontinence and therefore for urodynamic assessment, where this is indicated on other grounds.

Question D   1, 3 and 5 are correct.

Inflammation of the bladder mucosa may increase sensory input and so overcome cortical inhibition allowing uninhibited bladder contractions to occur and producing urge incontinence. Acute cystitis often presents in old people in this way. In such a case, the urinary tract infection should certainly be treated. However, many causes of incontinence are associated with a secondary infection which will not be successfully eradicated until the problem causing the incontinence has been removed. These include anatomical abnormalities of the bladder and urethra (e.g. calculi, diverticula) and residual urine. Often the residual urine is due to impaired bladder emptying in a neurogenic bladder and it is not possible to eliminate this. The continuing treatment of relapsing infection in these cases is not profitable or necessary.

In the present case, reinfection is most probable because of the regular soiling of the perineum with faeces. In such cases any attempt at prophylactic therapeutic treatment will only lead to the production of resistant organisms.

Question E

1. Imipramine may be effective in the uninhibited neurogenic bladder and unstable bladder because of its anticholinergic effect and several studies have shown it to be particularly useful in doses of 25 mg at night.

2. Occasionally faecal incontinence due to continuing diarrhoea in old people is directly due to bacterial overgrowth either at the upper end of the alimentary tract, in blind loops or diverticula, and possibly in this case, due to the effects of radiation. For this reason, a clinical trial with metronidazole may be worthwhile.

3. Methyl cellulose, by increasing the faecal bulk, may normalise the transit time and diminish diarrhoea. It is therefore worth a trial.

4. & 5.   Both codeine phosphate and phenoxylate hydrochloride are constipating agents and if the diarrhoea is intractable, as appears to be the case here, are worth a clinical trial.

Question F

In the present patient, because of the co-existence of urinary and faecal incontinence, none of the garments or pads suggested is likely to be very satisfactory.

In general, their advantages are as follows:

(a)   Kylie sheet - this has a non-wettable polyester sheet between the patient's skin and the absorbent part. The urine spreads fairly rapidly through the absorbent part and the patient's skin remains dry. The Kylie sheet is washable and trials have shown that it is reasonably effective in the management of urinary incontinence and that over a period of months it is much more cost effective than the use of disposable pads.

(b)   Maxi-plus pad with stretch knickers is a useful protective device for small and moderate quantities of urine. Stretch knickers, however, are difficult to put on with one hand and therefore of less use in stroke patients.

(c)   Kanga pants are of a polyester fabric and the pad is worn outside the pants in a waterproof cover pouch. The urine thus passes through the non-wettable fabric and is absorbed in the pad and the patient's skin remains dry. The pants come in many different types and sizes and must therefore be

161

carefully fitted, with the pad in direct apposition to the perineum. A disadvantage is the difficulty in removing the pad, which may be distasteful.

There may also be problems in disposing of pads from both types of body-worn appliances.

Question G   Either 1 or 3 may be correct.

The distinction between an unstable bladder and uninhibited neurogenic bladder is not generally agreed. Both of them may show the development of uninhibited contractions during bladder filling or alternatively as a result of provocation (e.g. standing or coughing). One generally accepted difference between these two conditions is that the unstable bladder is idiopathic whereas the uninhibited neurogenic bladder is associated with demonstrable disease in the central nervous system. However, this would not be apparent on the cystometrogram. The cystometrogram shown in Figure 14 has recordings from four channels. The top channel shows the rate and amount of filling, the second channel shows the pressure recorded from the bladder during filling, the lowest channel shows the pressure recorded from the rectum during filling, and the third channel (subtracted pressure) shows the bladder pressure minus the rectal pressure - that is the true pressure generated by the detrusor muscle.

The cystometrogram shows a large bladder contraction with 50 ml of filling, both with the patient lying and standing. The act of standing itself has not provoked a contraction, nor has coughing.

The series of waves shown in the lower three channels, particularly in the second half of the cystometrogram, has the appearance of transmitted pressure from periodic respiration which is more prominent in the rectum than in the bladder and is therefore still shown in the subtracted pressure.

Suggested further reading

Brocklehurst J C (1985) Ageing, bladder function and incontinence. In: Brocklehurst J C (ed.) Urology in the Elderly. Churchill Livingstone, Edinburgh

Robinson J M (1985) Evaluation of methods for assessment of bladder and urethral function. In: Brocklehurst J C (ed.) Urology in the Elderly. Churchill Livingstone, Edinburgh

CASE 30

PRESCRIBING FOR OLD PEOPLE

There is, perhaps, no subject in geriatric medicine of greater importance than the prescribing of drugs for the elderly; on the one hand the old receive more drugs than the young and often derive great benefit from them, while on the other hand, the old bear the major brunt of adverse drugs reactions (ADRs). In the UK the elderly receive approximately twice as many drugs as the national average, for example, 75% of persons over 75 years are taking one or more medicines at any one time. Among the elderly (>65 years) as a whole, 15% are taking a staggering four or more drugs at a time, and the very old (>85 years) are even more likely to be taking multiple drugs.

Question A

Which of the following statements are true about the consultation rate in general (family) practice in the UK?

1. Men over 75 years of age consult their family practitioner approximately:

    a)   once per annum

    b)   twice per annum

    c)   four times per annum

    d)   eight times per annum

    e)   16 times per annum

2. Women over the age of 75 years consult their family practitioner approximately:

    a)   once per annum

    b)   three times per annum

    c)   six times per annum

    d)   12 times per annum

    e)   18 times per annum

3. Old women consult their doctor more often than old men.

4. Old women consult their doctor more often than young women, but old men consult their doctor less often than young men.

163

Question B

Which of the following are true about adverse drug reactions (ADRs) in patients who are prescribed medication?

1. The incidence of ADRs in the very old (>85 years) is:

    a) 5%

    b) 10%

    c) 15%

    d) 20%

    e) 40%

2. The incidence of ADRs is higher in the UK than in the USA.

3. Of patients admitted to UK geriatric units, some are admitted solely or partially because of ADRs. This proportion is:

    a) 5%

    b) 10%

    c) 15%

    d) 20%

    e) 80%

4. Most ADRs are produced by drugs acting on the cardio-vascular or central nervous system.

5. Mental confusion is usually caused by drugs given for their sedative or anxiolytic effect, but may be caused by other drugs as well.

6. Falls in patients admitted to hospital are not uncommonly drug-induced.

Question C

Which of the following statements are true about drug disposition and action?

1. Pharmacodynamics is the study of drug absorption, distribution and elimination by the body.

2. Pharmacokinetic data from studies in the elderly are available for most drugs nowadays.

3. The old usually absorb less drug than the young when the drug is administered orally.

4. There is an increase in body water with age.

5. Hepatic handling of a drug is generally little changed in the elderly except for those drugs with a prominent "first pass" metabolism (high hepatic extraction).

6. Protein binding of drugs may be reduced in old patients.

7. Clinically significant reductions in the renal clearance of drugs (or their metabolites) in old people are not usually seen unless the blood urea (or creatinine) is raised, although minor reductions are occasionally seen in subjects with normal biochemical indices.

COMPLIANCE

Compliance may be defined as the extent to which the patient's behaviour coincides with the doctor's prescription.

Question D

1. "The elderly are generally less likely to comply with a prescription than the young" - true or false?

2. The proportion of the elderly on drugs who make errors in their compliance with prescriptions has been estimated to be:

   a) 10%

   b) 15%

   c) 25%

   d) 50%

   e) 75%

   f) 90%

3. The proportion of the elderly who make potentially serious errors in taking their medication is:

   a) 10%

   b) 15%

   c) 20%

   d) 25%

   e) 50%

   f) 75%

4. The number of different drugs normal old people can handle adequately has been shown to be:

   a) 2 drugs

   b) 3 drugs

   c) 4 drugs

   d) 5 drugs

   e) 6 drugs

   f) up to, but no more than, 10 drugs

5. Which of the following are generally regarded as factors in determining poor compliance in the elderly?

    a) Very old age (>85 years)

    b) Living alone

    c) Poor memory

    d) Poor understanding of the nature of the prescription

    e) Poor labelling of the drug container

    f) Difficulties in administration

6. Which of the following factors may help to improve patient compliance?

    a) Giving adequate information to the patient

    b) Using reasonable dosage regimens

    c) Using labelled "bubble packs" (single tablet bubbles)

    d) Restricting the number of different medications prescribed

    e) Providing written instructions

7. "Non-compliance is always harmful" - true or false?

DISCUSSION

Question A 1(a), 2(c), 3 are correct.

Unfortunately, the medical consultation rate does not parallel the increased prescription rate in the elderly. The consultation rate for elderly (>75 years) females is approximately six per annum, and the equivalent rate for elderly men is four per annum. The mean rates for all ages are approximately four and three per annum for women and men respectively. It is true that elderly women consult their doctor more than elderly men, but they are also prescribed more medication than men. The consultation rate for both elderly men and women is greater than other groups, but not in proportion to the increased prescription rate in the elderly age group. Thus, it appears that the elderly may have their prescriptions checked less often than the young, and this may be an important factor in drug problems in the elderly.

Question B 1(d), 2(b), 4, 5 and 6 are correct.

The number of ADRs rises with age because the proportion of the population taking drugs and the number of drugs taken rises with age, but also because the ADR rate in those on drugs rises with age (i.e. the old are more susceptible). Studies in different countries have shown an ADR rate of about 20% in 80-year-olds; the

166

rates in the UK and USA are similar. As a consequence of this high rate, about 10% of admissions to UK geriatric units are due to significant ADRs. Surveys have also shown that about two-thirds of all reactions are caused by drugs acting on the cardiovascular and central nervous systems. Non-steroidal anti-inflammatory agents (including aspirin), digoxin, and diuretics seem to be particularly common as a cause of life-threatening ADRs, probably because they are prescribed so frequently. Side-effects are often difficult to predict from a knowledge of the basic pharmacology of a drug; while most of the drugs causing confusion are obviously centrally acting, such as sedatives or tranquillisers, non-steroidal anti-inflammatory agents and histamine H2-receptor blockers may also cause confusion in the old. Thus, a high level of awareness is required in detecting ADRs as well as an adequate knowledge of previously recorded events.

A recent report on medication for the elderly identified five factors causing adverse reaction in the elderly: an inadequate clinical assessment; excessive prescribing; inadequate long-term supervision; altered pharmacokinetics and pharmacodynamics in the old; and problems with compliance. It is a basic principle of geriatric medicine that all patients need a thorough clinical assessment before a diagnosis can be made and treatment given. Although it seems natural to many to "spare the old" detailed investigation, the nature of disease in old age, and of the old themselves, often results in more investigations being needed to establish a diagnosis in the old than in younger patients. This is illustrated by the various cases in this book, and the point will not be further laboured here.

Question C   5 and 6 are correct.

Pharmacokinetics refers to the absorption, distribution and elimination of a drug by the body. Unfortunately, there is still little data available from experiments in the elderly. In the past, it has been customary to exclude the over 65s from drug studies, and although more elderly people are being studied (especially with new drugs), it is difficult to collect data from substantial numbers of the very old. It is a common mistake to lump all old people together; in general, the variance of any observation rises with age - what may be true at 65 is not likely to be true at 90. Some generalisations can be made about pharmacokinetics on the basis of known physiological changes with age; however, the pharmacodynamics of a drug (the body's response to a given drug concentration) may be more difficult to predict.

Most drugs are absorbed from the gastrointestinal tract to the same degree in young and old. However, absorption may be delayed, particularly when there is delayed gastric emptying which is a common accompaniment of severe illnesses. For this reason, initial doses of some antibiotics should be given parenterally in sick patients (e.g. those ill enough to be admitted to hospital). It should be borne in mind that absorption from intramuscular injection sites may be delayed (even more than oral absorption) in patients with circulatory failure. In these circumstances, intravenous injection should be considered.

There is little change in total body weight up to the sixth decade, and thereafter usually a slight decline. However, there is a 12% fall in total body water from maturity to old age, a marked rise in body fat (particularly in middle years) and a small decline in cell mass. These changes give rise to altered distribution spaces for various drugs (depending largely on their lipid solubility). In addition, there are alterations in plasma proteins (lower albumin, higher globulin) which may bind drugs; this may be particularly significant when several drugs which become protein bound are given at the same time. Thus, there are several factors which may alter the distribution of a drug within the body, and influence the free drug concentration at the tissue level. These changes are difficult to predict.

Many drugs are metabolised and inactivated in the liver (though the metabolites of several drugs - notably benzodiazepines - are also active and must be further excreted). Hepatic weight declines with age, and there are morphological changes in hepatocytes, and some biochemical alterations. However, in practice, changes in hepatic function do not seem to have striking effects on drug metabolism, and those which have been described are related to body weight, and may thus be allowed for if treatment is given on a "mg/kg" basis rather than a "mg/patient" basis. This is not true, however, for those drugs which have a prominent "first pass" metabolism in the liver (high hepatic extraction rates).

There is a steady (linear) and significant decline in cardiac output with age (about 1% per annum). This has important consequences for renal function but also possibly for drugs which are normally very avidly extracted by the liver. With such drugs (e.g. many β-adrenergic blockers, opiates, tricyclic anti-depressants and the sedative chlormethiazole) where the extraction rate is very high, the rate-limiting step is probably hepatic blood flow. Since hepatic blood flow declines with age (in hand with the fall in the cardiac output), it is not surprising that these drugs have a significantly longer half-life in the elderly, and also show higher peak plasma levels after a single oral dose. Any drug known to have a high extraction rate should thus be expected to have a greater effect in the elderly, and dosage should be adjusted accordingly.

While the changes described above may be important, they are overshadowed by the effects of declining renal function with age. This is further discussed in the section on "Interpreting routine biochemical profiles in old people", but a 60% reduction in the glomerular filtration rate should be anticipated by the age of 80 years. It is important to note that these changes are found in the well-elderly in addition to elderly patients. Furthermore, renal function is more difficult to calculate from the blood urea and creatinine than in younger patients (see section on "Interpreting routine biochemical profiles in old people"). Thus, if a drug is known to be largely renally excreted (e.g. digoxin) its dose should invariably be revised downwards when used in the elderly, although an accurate assessment of renal function may make dosage a less hit-and-miss affair. Nomograms for dosage with digoxin and gentamicin are available.

Thus, the pharmacokinetic data on the elderly suggests that, in general, the elderly need less of a drug for a given steady plasma concentration than the young. Two notable exceptions to this rule are tolbutamide and phenytoin, both of which have (normally) extensive protein binding. However, the reduction in dosage necessary for the elderly does not take into account altered tissue sensitivity to a given drug concentration (pharmacodynamics). Pharmacodynamic changes (sensitivity changes) may be in either direction, thus compounding the difficulty in predicting drug effects. For example, β-adrenergic receptors in the heart are either reduced in numbers with age, or reduced in sensitivity, thus a higher concentration of a β-agonist is required for an equivalent increase in heart rate and conversely, a higher dose of a β-blocker may be required for the same blockade. So with regard to propranolol, the pharmacokinetic alterations which give rise to a higher blood concentration for a given oral dose are partially offset by reduced cardiac sensitivity to this drug. Conversely, the increased sensitivity to the central action of benzodiazepines compounds the reduced clearance of this class of drugs.

Question D   2(e), 3(a), 4(b), 5(a-e) and 6(a,b,d,e) are correct.

Compliance with drug therapy has been shown to be poor at all ages, and the elderly, as a whole, are probably no worse in this regard than younger patients; indeed, for certain classes of medication, the elderly may be more compliant than the young. Nevertheless, it has been estimated that 75% of old people make mistakes (usually omissions) in taking their drugs, and in 20% these mistakes may be potentially serious. In addition, there is a subgroup of elderly patients in whom compliance may be particularly poor, or particularly dangerous, because of multiple prescribing and multiple pathology. Very old patients (>85 years), living alone and with poor memory, are particularly at risk. Non-compliance is commonly due to failure to understand the nature of the medication, and to inadequate instructions and labelling on the drug container itself. Surprisingly, difficulty with administration, swallowing or unpleasant flavour are not usually a cause of failure to attempt to take a treatment. Oesophageal motility problems are common in the elderly, and studies have shown prolonged retention of tablets and capsules in the lower oesophagus. Patients should be encouraged to take their tablets with liberal fluids. An inadequate physical technique, such as with metered dose inhalers, while not reducing the frequency of administration, may lead to an ineffective dose being delivered. Again, this problem is not confined to the old. It should be noted, however, that the old often have difficulty using "child-proof" containers and "blister packs" which perhaps should not be routinely issued to this age group.

It has been repeatedly shown that normal old people can only reliably handle up to three separate medications daily and regimens of administration may have to be kept simple in order not to exceed this. For example, once or twice daily (only) dosage should be aimed for, the use of combined preparations should be considered where appropriate, or even intermittent injection (for example, vitamin D) in place of adding yet another tablet to a long list. The importance of providing clear written instruction cannot be over-emphasised, and all prescribers should test their patients in order to check that information has been correctly registered in the first place. Instructions may well have to be repeated.

Non-compliance is not always harmful, and all geriatricians can recount cases where ADRs have only occurred after admission to hospital, when an unreasonable drug load has been faithfully administered by the nursing staff. As at any age, if a reasonable prescribed dose is not having the effect you expect, consider that the medication is probably not being taken, and do not slavishly prescribe a higher dose. Drug levels (particularly of digoxin and anti-convulsants) may be very helpful in this situation.

Good prescribing habits should be learned before qualification and are important in all branches of medicine; nevertheless the following ten points are offered as a summary of good practice with particular regard to the elderly.

TEN RULES FOR DRUG PRESCRIBING IN THE ELDERLY

1. Always try to make a DIAGNOSIS before prescribing, rather than just treating symptoms; consider carefully if treatment is really NECESSARY and SAFE, and formulate a clear MANAGE-MENT plan.

2. Only use drugs YOU KNOW, particularly with regard to their pharmacokinetics and side-effects. Make your choice in the light of OTHER MEDICATION being received by the patient (remember they may be receiving drugs from elsewhere), and OTHER ILLNESSES present.

3. Select an APPROPRIATE DOSE for your elderly subject, making use of nomograms, renal function tests, etc. if necessary.

4. Use the SIMPLEST POSSIBLE REGIMEN OF ADMINISTRATION, sticking to once daily doses if possible.

5. EXPLAIN the object and the nature of treatment to the patient and anyone else who may be treating or caring for the patient. Give CLEAR, WRITTEN INSTRUCTIONS,and expect to have to repeat them.

6. Make a definite PLAN to REVIEW PROGRESS (to see whether your objects have been achieved) and ALL MEDICATION (to ensure nothing has changed), and to check COMPLIANCE.

7. Do not allow elderly patients to DEFAULT; they may be unable to attend because of illness, for example an adverse drug reaction that you have caused.

8. STOP medication shown to be INEFFECTIVE and RECORD the facts so that others (or even yourself) will not repeat the prescription fruitlessly. REPORT all (suspected) adverse reactions to the appropriate authority (Committee on Safety of Medicines, in the UK).

9. Consider before STOPPING someone else's prescription that good reasons may have existed for it to have been started, but which are not obvious to you; make careful ENQUIRIES. STOPPING medication may require as careful a MANAGEMENT PLAN as starting it.

10. Remember that NO MEDICAL CONSULTATION with an elderly patient is COMPLETE until ALL DRUGS and the PRESCRIPTION SHEET have been carefully reviewed.

Suggested further reading

O'Malley K (ed.) (1984) Clinical Pharmacology and Drug Treatment in the Elderly. Churchill Livingstone, Edinburgh

Royal College of Physicians (1984) Medication for the elderly. Journal of the Royal College of Physicians (London), 18, 3-10

CASE 31

BONE PAIN

HISTORY AND EXAMINATION

A 72-year-old man living alone has had osteoarthritis of his right knee since an injury many years previously. Now this makes him housebound and dependent on a neighbour for shopping. He also has meals-on-wheels three times a week as his main source of cooked food although he does make snacks for himself. He is being treated with non-steroidal anti-inflammatory drugs which he has been taking for some years and this has kept his pain reasonably at bay although his mobility has been limited also by a degree of flexion contracture of the right knee. However, in the last two years the pain in the leg has been increasing and he has also complained of some pain in the left leg and of low back ache.

ON EXAMINATION

He is a thin and undernourished-looking man. There is destructive arthritis of the right knee with a flexion deformity of 20° short of full extension. There is marked muscle wasting in the thigh and the left femur is very prominent. It feels hotter than the right. In fact, the pain he describes is in the upper and middle thigh and in the back. The bones are not tender. Reflexes are present and plantars flexor. He has a moderate kyphosis and some limitation of lumbar flexion and extension. He also has a palpable liver.

Question A

What is the differential diagnosis?

Question B

What investigations are required and for what reason?

INVESTIGATIONS

A biochemical profile is normal except for:

Serum calcium (2.70 mmol/l)

Serum alkaline phosphatase (450 iu/l)

Serum albumin (30 g/l)

Serum globulin (38.5 g/l)

According to Hodkinson's nomogram (Hodkinson, 1977) the corrected calcium with these findings is 1.6 mmol/l which is slightly higher than the normal range (1.3-1.5). An isoenzyme study indicated that the alkaline phosphatase derives from bone.

Rectal examination showed a moderately enlarged smooth and firm prostate.

X-ray of the pelvis is shown in Figure 15.

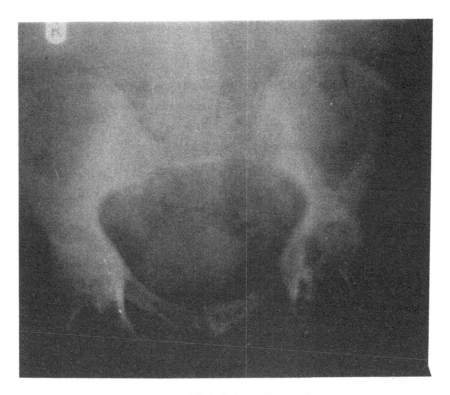

Figure 15 Pelvic radiograph

Question C

Which of the following symptoms may be caused by Paget's disease?

1.　　Mental confusion

2.　　Haematuria

3.　　Proximal myopathy

4.　　Dysarthria

5.　　Urinary incontinence

Question D

Pain in Paget's disease may be due to:

1.   Associated osteoarthritis

2.   Trabecular fracture

3.   Increased blood supply

4.   Stretching of the periosteum

5.   Muscle spasm

Question E

Deafness as a result of Paget's disease may be due to:

1.   Impaired circulation through the cochlear artery

2.   Involvement of the stapes in the disease

3.   Damage to the auditory nerve by stretching

4.   Involvement of the cochlea in the disease

5.   Wax in the ears

Question F

Write brief notes on the following in the treatment of Paget's disease:

1.   Fluoride

2.   Calcitonin

3.   Mithramycin

4.   Sodium etidronate

ANSWERS

Question A Differential diagnosis

1.   Paget's disease. The hot non-tender shaft of femur which he indicated as the centre of the pain, and the pain not being relieved by non-steroidal anti-inflammatory drugs, are highly suggestive of Paget's disease.

2.   Osteoarthritis and spondylosis. Osteoarthritis of the knee with deformity and flexion contracture may have led to pelvic tilt and lumbar spondylosis with osteophytes. These could produce low back pain and referred pain (sciatica).

3.   Osteomalacia. Bone pain and back pain may be presenting symptoms of osteomalacia; this should be suspected especially in someone who has a poor diet. If the pain is severe then the bones may be tender.

174

4. Secondary carcinoma. Metastases from carcinoma of the prostate are common in the pelvis and femora and may produce a
clinical picture similar to that described here. The palpable
liver may indicate metastases although this is not a usual site
from prostatic carcinoma.

5. Multiple myeloma. Bony deposits tend to begin centrally and
may involve the pelvis and the upper end of the femora at an
early stage. The majority of cases present with bone pain.

6. Osteoporosis. This is unlikely to produce pain in the thighs
and is less common in males.

7. Hyperparathyroidism producing osteitis fibrosis cystica is a
possibility.

Question B

1. Rectal examination is essential to exclude carcinoma of the
prostate.

2. X-rays of the legs, pelvis and lumbar spine. These will
clearly distinguish Paget's disease, bony metastases (which
from prostatic carcinoma may be sclerotic), multiple myeloma
and in the presence of osteomalacia, may indicate Looser's
zones (pseudo-fractures). X-ray of the lumbar spine may
indicate any of these diseases and there will almost certainly
be marked osteophytosis in view of the deformity of the right
knee.

3. Biochemistry. A normal urea and creatinine help to rule out
renal failure and this is important since impaired renal function might reduce the amount by which the serum phosphate is
lowered in hyperparathyroidism. The key investigation, of
course, is the highly elevated alkaline phosphatase of bone
type. This indicates osteoblastic activity and is very high in
Paget's disease although it may also be elevated in osteomalacia and metastases.

   Serum calcium may be normal or slightly elevated in
Paget's disease. It may be elevated in multiple myeloma. A
marked elevation is more likely to indicate hyperparathyroidism. The corrected calcium (corrected for serum
albumin level which is often low in old people) may be more
useful if there is any doubt. The corrected level here is
slightly elevated and in keeping with the diagnosis of Paget's
disease. In osteomalacia, of course, the calcium would be normal or low.

   Serum phosphate would be normal in all these diseases
except for osteomalacia and hyperparathyroidism in which it
may be diminished, though serum phosphate is not useful in
screening biochemically for osteomalacia in old people.

   Serum acid phosphatase is occasionally elevated in
Paget's disease but high levels are characteristic of prostatic

175

carcinoma, either from the lesion within the prostate (it is produced by prostatic epithelium) or from the bone, where it is a manifestation of osteoclastic activity.

The presence of hepatic disease could, of course, account for the changes in plasma proteins and alkaline phosphatase, though this is greater than would be expected with liver disease and the isoenzyme test indicates it is not of hepatic origin.

4. A technetium bone scan is a possible investigation if there is any doubt as to the presence of metastases but in this case with radiological evidence of Paget's disease it would be inappropriate.

5. Urinary hydroxyproline is another possible test which would be elevated in Paget's disease but in this patient it is not necessary.

Question C   1, 2, 4 and 5 are correct.

All but number 3 (proximal myopathy) may be caused by Paget's disease. Mental confusion and dysarthria may both result from platybasia (with basilar compression). Urinary incontinence may indicate spinal cord compression and haematuria may be a manifestation of urinary calculus. Proximal myopathy is not a feature of Paget's disease and is characteristic of osteomalacia.

Question D   1, 2, 3 and 4 are correct.

Pain receptors in bone are present in the periosteum and in the blood vessels and direct bony pain may result from stretching of the periosteum or of the blood spaces. It may also result from trabecular fractures. Paget's disease is also associated with a form of osteoarthritis in nearby joints and this also may be a factor in producing pain.

Question E   2, 3 and 4 are correct.

Wax may co-exist with Paget's disease and impair hearing but is not directly caused by the disease. The blood supply is not usually impaired. The Pagetic process in the temporal bone may breach the endolymph surface of the cochlea. The auditory nerve may be stretched and the ossicles may be affected by the disease.

Question F

1. Fluoride - this has been used in the past in the treatment of Paget's disease with some improvement. However, the toxic effects are considerable and it is no longer in general use.

2. Calcitonin is generally regarded as the treatment of choice at present. It inhibits the activity of osteoclasts and its results

are demonstrable radiologically. Its principal effect is to reduce pain but it has also been shown to provide some improvement in neurological complications. It may produce complete biochemical and clinical remission, or improvement without the biochemical values returning to complete normality: about 50% decrease in serum alkaline phosphatase and urinary hydroxyproline occurs. The drug is rarely toxic apart from mild side-effects. It may, however, induce antibody formation with consequent resistance to its action. It is usually given for up to six months but if a clinical effect is not apparent within the first two months then it should not be persisted with. One disadvantage is that it has to be given sub-cutaneously.

3. Mythramycin - a cytotoxic drug - is given intravenously and has a toxic effect on osteoclasts. However, it has much more potentially dangerous side-effects than the others and its use is therefore limited in Paget's disease although its effects may be dramatic.

4. Diphosphonates - these may be given orally or by intravenous injection. They retard the precipitation of calcium phosphate from solution and also reduce bone resorption. In the wrong dose, however, they may make bone pain worse and some worsening has been noted radiologically. The generally used drug is etidronate disodium and the more recently produced APD. Diphosphonates may be required for up to six months before an effect becomes apparent and the remission thereafter may be prolonged to a year or more. However, high doses have recently been shown to be effective within one month.

Suggested further reading

Handy R C (1981) Paget's Disease of Bone: Assessment and Management. Praeger, Eastbourne

Hodkinson H M (1977) Biochemical Diagnosis of the Elderly, p.55. Chapman and Hall, London

Preston C J, Yates A J P, Beneton M N C, Russell R G G, Gray R E S, Smith R and Kanis J A (1986) Effective short term treatment of Paget's disease with oral etidronate. British Medical Journal, 282, 79-80

CASE 32

INTERPRETING ROUTINE BIOCHEMICAL PROFILES IN OLD PEOPLE

Investigation of patients by the routine use of a multichannel biochemical autoanalyser has become commonplace. It is important to assess the significance of the "profile" of results generated by this method, bearing in mind that if the normal range is defined as composed of 95% of the healthy population, then the probability of generating a completely "normal" profile is 0.95 x (the number of independent tests), so if there are 12 independent tests, about half of the people will show at least one "abnormality" and if one considers only abnormalities in one direction (e.g. raised levels only), about a quarter will be abnormal. These considerations do not differ for the elderly, but since the normal ranges of certain tests are slightly different in the old, erroneous conclusions can be drawn if ranges relevant to a younger population are applied. This is of particular importance in assessing renal function and diagnosing osteomalacia.

Question A

Which of the following are true about biochemical findings in the elderly?

1. Hyponatraemia is commonly due to diuretics.

2. The serum potassium will fall below 3.5 mmol/l in the majority of old people given a loop diuretic unless they are given a potassium supplement or a potassium-sparing agent, such as spironolactone.

3. The serum albumin and globulin fall slightly with age.

4. The commonest cause of a raised alkaline phosphatase among the elderly is gall stones, followed by osteomalacia.

5. The serum phosphate is usually low in elderly patients with osteomalacia.

6. For routine purposes, the glomerular filtration rate can be assessed from the serum creatinine, body weight and age.

7. L-dopa may interfere with thyroid function tests.

ANSWERS AND DISCUSSION

Question A   1, 6 and 7 are correct.

Proteins

Albumin   There is probably a slight decrease in serum albumin in well old people; significant hypoalbuminaemia is comparatively common in acutely ill elderly patients. As well as being a marker for the severity of a constitutional disorder, the fall in serum albumin has implications for the diagnosis of osteomalacia (see below) and the use of drugs which are protein-bound in the circulation (see section on "Prescribing for Old People").

Globulins   The major change in the globulin fraction in the old is due to a significant rise in IgG levels; this in turn has been postulated to be due to a lower activity of T-suppressor cells (T-lymphocytes with suppressor activity) in old people. Most routine analyses measure the total protein, and the albumin (by a dye binding method) and compute the "globulin" by subtraction of the albumin from the total protein. This "globulin" measurement thus includes a wide variety of proteins, the major constituents of which, apart from immuno-globulins, are ovosomucoid (which shows little change with age), thromboglobulin and hepatoglobulin (which increase with age) and transferrin (which shows a slight decrease with age).

Alkaline phosphatase   It is as well to remember that the commonest cause of a raised alkaline phosphatase in the elderly is Paget's disease of the bone. Most cases can be diagnosed with a plain radiograph of the chest and pelvis, although no bone is immune and skull involvement is not rare. Minor changes in the alkaline phosphatase are common in elderly patients and are often ignored. It is, however, an important marker for osteomalacia (see below).

Electrolytes (Sodium, potassium, chloride and bicarbonate)

These have exactly the same significance as in the young. Note the following points:

Sodium   Severe hyponatraemia (<125 mmol/l) is present in about 5% of acutely ill old people, and is commonly due to diuretics.

Potassium   There is a small decline in total body potassium with age, consistent with the fall in cell mass with age; the serum potassium is unaffected. Most old people do not develop a low serum potassium when taking diuretics. Those that do usually show a fall in the serum potassium in the early weeks of treatment. Remember that sustained release potassium tablets commonly lodge in the lower oesophagus of elderly people and may cause ulceration. They only contain 8 mmol/l of potassium which is about the same as a cup of coffee (5 mmol/l of potassium per teaspoon of instant coffee).

Calcium and phosphate

Osteomalacia is common in patients with fractured neck of femur (perhaps being present in 30% of cases) and, to a mild degree, in those who are housebound. Florid osteomalacia is rare. An oral intake of vitamin D of about 100 iu/day is known to prevent rickets in children, but the majority of vitamin D is synthesised in the skin by the action of sunlight. The old commonly have oral intakes of less than 100 iu of vitamin D daily; they have lower serum vitamin D levels than the young , and if unable to gain sufficient sunlight exposure, are at high risk from developing osteomalacia.

Serum phosphate levels are partially dependent on renal function, and the fall in glomerular filtration rate with age leads to a rise in the serum phosphate. This test is thus of poor discriminant value in the diagnosis of osteomalacia. Only about 50% of the total serum calcium is free, the major binding being to albumin, and to a lesser extent, globulin, and complex formation with other ions. A correction should be applied to the total serum calcium for this, and a formula for computing the corrected free calcium from albumin and globulin measurements has been published and validated in elderly patients. The finding of a low "corrected" calcium should prompt a search for Looser's zones if the alkaline phosphatase is high, and in the housebound elderly is probably sufficient justification for vitamin D supplements (400 iu/day) to be given. Minor degrees of hypocalcaemia may be missed, particularly in subjects with a normal albumin and a high globulin, unless a correction is made.

Blood urea and creatinine

There is a linear decline in the glomerular filtration rate (GFR) with age of approximately 1 ml/min/year (after the age of 20 years). In younger patients, the GFR can be shown to be inversely proportional to the blood urea and creatinine measurements; thus a halving of the GFR is associated with a doubling of the serum creatinine. In the old, however, there is a decline in protein intake which tends to reduce the blood urea, and a decline in muscle mass, which tends to reduce the serum creatinine. Thus, it is not uncommon to find frail elderly subjects with a GFR (measured from the endogenous creatinine clearance) of only 20-30 ml/min, with the blood urea and creatinine well within the normal range. In one study of patients with a serum creatinine of less than 125 μmol/l, the creatinine clearances varied from a mean of 110 ml/min in 20-year-olds, 64 ml/min in 70-year-olds, 47 ml/min in 80-year-olds, to 34 ml/min in 90-year-olds. Thus, age and weight must be taken into account when estimating the GFR from either urea or creatinine.

Nomograms enabling this to be done at the bedside have been published, and are particularly helpful when prescribing drugs which are predominantly excreted by the kidneys.

Suggested further reading

Hodkinson M (ed.) (1984) Clinical Biochemistry of the Elderly. Churchill Livingstone, Edinburgh

Sievsback-Nielson K et al (1971) Rapid evaluation of creatinine clearance. Lancet, 1, 1133-1134

CASE 33

CONFUSION AND
LOSS OF APPETITE

An 80-year-old widower was one day found by his sister to be irritable and confused. He refused food and complained vaguely of a pain in the right side of his chest. The next day he was much the same, and he had been restless throughout the night. He had smoked cigarettes for most of his life and had a daily cough with sputum.

He fell to the floor and was unable to rise, an ambulance was called and he was admitted to hospital as an urgency.

It was impossible to obtain much of a history from either the patient or his sister. His general practitioner thought he was taking no drugs. Physical examination showed a perplexed, fidgety man who was disorientated in time and place. Pulse 96, regular, blood pressure 160/85 mmHg, respiratory rate 32/minute, there were coarse crepitations at both lung bases. His sublingual temperature was 37.3°C. There were no other findings of importance.

Question A

Comment on the temperature.

Question B

What is the most likely diagnosis and which investigations would you perform as soon as possible?

Question C

Comment on the chest radiograph in Figure 16.

Question D

List the evidence in favour of the diagnosis of pneumonia.

Question E

Which of the following are true?

1. Most elderly patients with pneumonia have respiratory symptoms.

2. Pneumococcal pneumonia is rare in old age.

3. More than 50% of elderly patients with pneumonia are afebrile at the time of presentation.

182

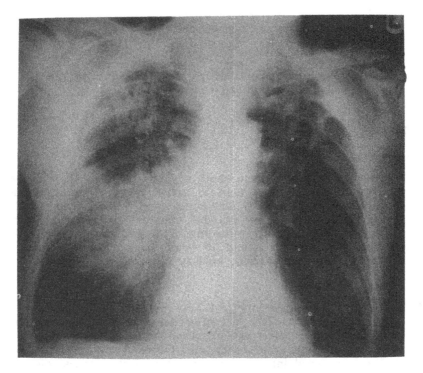

Figure 16 Chest radiograph

4. The chest radiograph is often still abnormal four weeks after treatment for pneumonia in patients over 70 years old.

5. More than half of the cases of pneumonia acquired in long-stay geriatric wards and nursing homes are caused by Gram-negative bacteria.

Question F

True or false?

Mortality in elderly patients with acute consolidating pneumonia:

1. Is not related to the PaO$_2$ at the time of admission to hospital.

2. The fatality rate is less than 10% when appropriate antibiotic treatment is given.

3. The fatality rate is higher in patients who are confused at the time of admission.

4. The fatality rate is higher in bacteraemic patients.

5. The overall fatality rate is about 80% in the ninth decade irrespective of treatment.

Question G

Why are old people so prone to pneumonia?

Question H

Describe measures which might reduce the attack rate of pneumonia in relatively well old people living at home.

ANSWERS

Question A

Sublingual temperature measurements are unreliable in the elderly, mainly because the patients tend to mouth breath when they are tachypnoeic (as in this case) and hence tend to cool their mouth. Since the core temperature will be underestimated under these circumstances, a sublingual recording of 37.3°C suggests that the patient could be pyrexial, and it would be advisable to take a rectal, or 5-minute, supervised, axillary temperature.

Question B

The combination of an acute confusional state, tachypnoea and pyrexia should always alert the physician to the probable diagnosis of pneumonia, though other conditions, for example, pulmonary embolism and myocardial infarction can cause a similar clinical picture, including a low grade fever.

     The essential investigation is a chest radiograph. Also, arterial blood gases should be measured; patients are often more hypoxic than is clinically apparent, and may require oxygen supplementation. A white blood cell count, if markedly raised, supports the diagnosis of infection. An ECG will help to rule out myocardial infarction, and may give evidence of a pulmonary embolus.

Question C

The chest radiograph shows an area of patchy consolidation in the right mid-zone. The appearance is suggestive (but not diagnostic) of acute pyogenic pneumonia. The heart size is normal, so heart failure and pulmonary embolism are less likely as diagnoses. Old TB scarring can be seen at the apices.

Question D

Features which support the diagnosis of pneumonia are the chest radiograph appearance, the probable fever, the acute onset of a confusional state, the preceding history of chronic bronchitis due to cigarette smoking and the tachypnoea. The chest pain was possibly pleuritic.

184

The bilateral coarse basal lung crepitations contribute virtually nothing to the diagnosis, as they are frequently found in chronic bronchitis, and are often noticed in well old people.

Question E 4 and 5 are true.

While it is true to say that some elderly patients with pneumonia have no respiratory symptoms, the majority do. Furthermore, the more carefully the physician extracts the history in such cases, the more respiratory symptoms of a relatively subtle nature will emerge, such as a fall in exercise tolerance or recent slight cough. Confused old people are usually uncertain of their symptoms, though they may have complained to relatives who can then convey the symptoms to the physician second hand.

Pneumococcal pneumonia is not rare in old people; in some surveys of community acquired pneumonia, it ranks as one of the highest as a cause of acute bacterial pneumonia.

Recent evidence suggests that most old people mount a febrile response to infection. In the past, the belief that many old people remain afebrile when infected has probably been largely due to inaccurate temperature measurement techniques, which do not detect the often mild pyrexia that seems to occur in the old. Also, antibiotics given before admission to hospital render many patients genuinely afebrile.

The radiographic changes of pneumonia take longer to resolve in old age; it is not uncommon for residual shadowing to be present up to 6 weeks after an acute pneumonia. If the patient is constitutionally well, the temptation to give repeated courses of antibiotics must be resisted.

Gram-negative organisms have a predilection to cause lower respiratory tract infection in frail debilitated old people, and the long-stay hospital environment always has such organisms present. Hence the very high incidence of Gram-negative pneumonia in nursing homes and continuing care wards. Excessive colonisation of the oropharynx and upper respiratory tract with these organisms in the debilitated elderly with a tendency to aspirate oral secretions, is the likely precursor to these pneumonias.

Question F 3, 4 and 5 are true.

Recent evidence shows that hypoxia is strongly predicative of mortality in old people with pneumonia; the mortality is very high in those with PaO_2 of less than 7 kPa when breathing air at the time of admission to hospital.

The fatality rate of people with pneumonia aged 70 years and above is much higher than that of young adults. Most surveys indicate that over 25% will die despite appropriate treatment.

Confusion indicates a poorer prognosis in pneumonia in old age; this is probably closely related to the poor prognosis associated with hypoxia.

Bacteraemia probably reflects the intensity of bacterial proliferation in pneumonia and is associated with a poorer prognosis in most surveys. This is particularly true when Gram-negative pneumonia is associated with the presence of Gram-negative organisms in the blood; the mortality rate has been 100% in some studies.

The older the patient the higher the likelihood of death during an episode of pneumonia. Generally, the overall mortality is less than 10% in the third decade, rising to about 30% in the sixth decade, and 80% in the ninth decade.

Question G

Many factors contribute to the proneness of old people to pneumonia. These are summarised in Figure 17, and a hypothetical sequence of events leading to pneumonia in the debilitated elderly is shown in Figure 18.

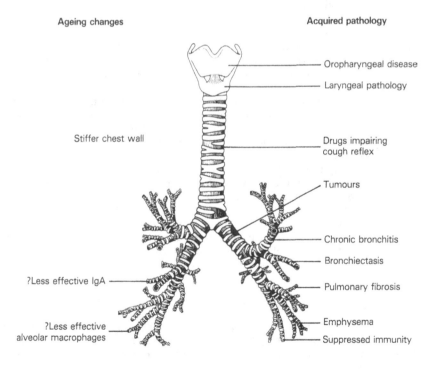

Ageing changes

Acquired pathology

Oropharyngeal disease

Laryngeal pathology

Stiffer chest wall

Drugs impairing
cough reflex

Tumours

Chronic bronchitis

Bronchiectasis

?Less effective IgA

Pulmonary fibrosis

?Less effective
alveolar macrophages

Emphysema

Suppressed immunity

Figure 17 Factors predisposing to pneumonia in old age

Question H

There are a number of measures which might reduce the risk of pneumonia in an elderly individual who is in reasonably good health. Stopping smoking and moderation in the use of alcohol are both

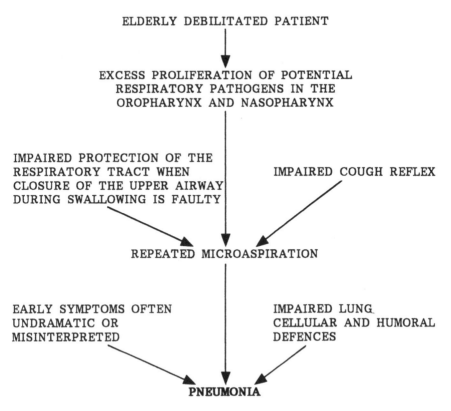

Figure 18 Hypothetical sequence of events leading to pneumonia in the debilitated elderly patient

important. Adequate heating to reduce the risk of pneumonia as a consequence of hypothermia, an adequate diet and avoidance of dehydration are all worthwhile. There is fairly good evidence that influenza and pneumococcal vaccines can reduce the attack rate of pneumonia, though the protection is by no means perfect. Prompt treatment of infective exacerbations of chronic bronchitis helps prevent these becoming frank consolidating pneumonias. Drugs which impair the cough reflex or lower the level of consciousness should be used with caution. Any measures which reduce the likelihood of falls will help, since old people who are unable to rise from the floor are predisposed to pneumonia.

Although hard evidence is lacking, it appears likely that poor dental hygiene and ill-fitting dentures might increase the risk of pneumonia by encouraging the overgrowth of respiratory pathogens in the mouth; it is probably worthwhile advising such patients to seek dental advice for that reason.

Suggested further reading

Elbright J R, Rytel M W (1980) Bacterial pneumonia in the elderly. *Journal of the American Geriatrics Society*, **28**, 220-223

Freeman E (1985) The respiratory system. In: Brocklehurst J C (ed.) *Textbook of Geriatric Medicine and Gerontology*, 3rd Edn. Churchill Livingstone, Edinburgh

READING LIST

GENERAL REFERENCE

1. Brocklehurst J C (ed.) (1985) <u>Textbook of Geriatric Medicine and Gerontology</u>, 3rd Edn. Churchill Livingstone, Edinburgh

2. Exton-Smith A N and Weksler M E (eds.) (1985) <u>Practical Geriatric Medicine</u>, Churchill Livingstone, Edinburgh

3. Anderson F and Williams B (1983) <u>Practical Management of the Elderly</u>, Black-wells, Oxford

4. Hamdy R C (1984) <u>Geriatric Medicine. A Problem-Orientated Approach</u>, Balliere Tindall, London

5. Ham R J (ed.) (1983) <u>Primary Care Geriatrics. A Case-Based Learning Program</u>, John Wright PSG Inc.

6. Thompson M K (1984) <u>The Care of the Elderly in General Practice</u>, Churchill Livingstone, Edinburgh

7. Brocklehurst J C and Allen S C (1987) <u>Geriatric Medicine for Students</u>, 3rd Edn. Churchill Livingstone, Edinburgh

SERVICES AND ORGANISATION

1. Isaacs B and Evers H (eds.) (1984) <u>Innovation in the Care of the Elderly</u>, Croom Helm, Beckenham

2. Lishman J and Horobin G (eds.) (1985) <u>Developing Services for the Elderly</u>, Kogan Page, London

3. Gilleard C J. (1984) <u>Living with Dementia: Community Care of the Elderly Mentally Infirm</u>, Croom Helm, Beckenham

4. Skeet M. (1983) <u>Protecting the Health of the Elderly: A Review of WHO Activities</u>, HMSO Publications, London

SELECTED MONOGRAPHS

1. Hodkinson H M (ed.) (1984) <u>Clinical Biochemistry in the Elderly</u>, Churchill Livingstone, Edinburgh

2. Paterson C R and MacLennan W J (1984) <u>Bone Disease in the Elderly</u>, John Wiley, Chichester

3. Wright V (ed.) (1983) <u>Bone and Joint Disease in the Elderly</u>, Churchill Livingstone, Edinburgh

4. Fox R A (ed.) (1984) <u>Immunology and Infection in the Elderly</u>, Churchill Livingstone, Edinburgh

5. Stout R W (ed.) (1984) <u>Arterial Disease in the Elderly</u>, Churchill Livingstone, Edinburgh

6. Stott N C H and Finlay I G (1984) <u>Care of the Dying</u>, Churchill Livingstone, Edinburgh

7. Hellemans J and Vantrappen G (eds.) (1984) <u>Gastrointestinal Tract Disorders in the Elderly</u>, Churchill Livingstone, Edinburgh

8. Brocklehurst J C (ed.) (1984) <u>Urology in the Elderly</u>, Churchill Livingstone, Edinburgh

9. Mulley G P (1984) <u>Practical Management of Stroke</u>, Croom Helm, Beckenham

INDEX